# The Writing Warrior

## Also by Laraine Herring

### NONFICTION

*Writing Begins with the Breath: Embodying Your Authentic Voice*
*Lost Fathers: How Women Can Heal from Adolescent Father Loss*

### FICTION

*Ghost Swamp Blues*
*Monsoons: A Collection of Writing*

# *The* Writing Warrior

## DISCOVERING THE COURAGE TO FREE YOUR TRUE VOICE

Laraine Herring

SHAMBHALA
Boston & London
2010

Shambhala Publications, Inc.
Horticultural Hall
300 Massachusetts Avenue
Boston, Massachusetts 02115
www.shambhala.com

9 8 7 6 5 4 3 2 1

First Edition
Printed in the United States of America

∞ This edition is printed on acid-free paper that meets the
American National Standards Institute z39.48 Standard.
♻ This book was printed on 30% postconsumer recycled paper.
For more information please visit www.shambhala.com.
Distributed in the United States by Random House, Inc., and
in Canada by Random House of Canada Ltd

Interior design and composition: Greta D. Sibley & Associates

Library of Congress Cataloging-in-Publication Data

Herring, Laraine, 1968–
The writing warrior: discovering the courage to free your true voice /
Laraine Herrring.—1st ed.
p. cm.
ISBN 978-1-59030-796-0 (pbk.: alk. paper)
1. Authorship—Psychological aspects. I. Title.
PN171.P83H475 2010
808'.02019—dc22
2010008804

*for Jeffrey Hartgraves*
*1961–2008*
*ciao*

# Contents

*Contents*

PART THREE: Dissolving Your Illusions

PART FOUR: Committing to Your Authentic Path

# Acknowledgments

Gayle Brandeis: for being my first reader, my deepest reader, and the companion of my writer's heart.

Cain Carroll: for teaching me to stand steady without sticking.

Keith Haynes: for being present and helping me soften and open.

Linda Roghaar: for unflappable belief in my work.

Jennifer Urban-Brown: for faith in my writing and a brilliant editing of this manuscript.

Alma Luz Villanueva: for embodying the writing warrior so I could one day see it in myself.

My parents, Glenn and Elinor Herring, who taught me to be fierce and fearless.

And finally, my students, without whom I would have learned nothing.

# Introduction

> To change skins, evolve into new cycles, I feel one
> has to learn to discard. If one changes internally,
> one should not continue to live with the same
> objects. They reflect one's mind and the psyche of
> yesterday. I throw away what has no dynamic, liv-
> ing use.
>
> —Anaïs Nin

I taught writing long before I truly believed I was a writer. Fortunately, I learned a few things quickly in the class-room. One: teaching is hard. Two: teaching keeps you in the moment. And three: I love to teach. These three pieces of information begged the next logical question: did I have anything to teach? Most of my students were decades older than me. I had some publishing credits, but not many. I was young and looked younger. I had enough arrogance and ego to act like I'd done it a million times before. And, fortunately, enough awareness to know I had no idea what I was doing.

During my second year of teaching, I taught creative writing classes during the evenings, while still working full time and attending graduate school. I had learned early, thankfully, the first rule of effective teaching: talk less, listen more.

I didn't yet know that was a foundation for writing as well. I began to notice that even though I was teaching fiction, my students were writing their lives, loosely disguised with fictional places or times. They were writing their fears, their obsessions, and their wounds in black and white on twenty-pound bond paper, but many of them didn't know it. Many of them believed they were indeed making everything up. They believed there was nothing of themselves in these men and women who peopled their work.

For the first time, I began to understand the courage and absolute vulnerability it took to put words on a page. It was no more or less courageous if the author didn't know what she or he was doing. *The work knew what it was doing.* The more their work came from their brains, the less effective it was. The more they planned, the less they grew. Students outed themselves in their stories. They wrote themselves into their own sexuality without trying. They longed for the absent love of a mother or mourned the loss of a child. They wrote and rewrote mistakes of their past trying to find a different ending. They showed me that writing is not a series of ingredients (character + plot + dialogue + setting + conflict) placed in a particular predetermined Aristotelian order. Writing was alive. Through writing, the writers became electric.

"You are writing warriors," I said one day in class, and we growled and made warrior sounds until we laughed. "You have no idea how brave you are." And they looked at me with open, surprised eyes, their brains not quite grasping what I was saying, but their hearts responding. Message received.

In *Writing Begins with the Breath,* I wanted to give people an opportunity to view the writing process as something more than a series of steps one could cross off a list. I hoped to expand writing for the reader. Put it on a cellular level. Expand it like the belly on an inhale. And most of all, I hoped to surprise people by the ease with which they could contact themselves through writing if they opened up channels within themselves to listen.

When thinking of the next step after *Writing Begins with the Breath,* I returned to that first moment of bravery required to expose yourself on the page and the first moment I learned not just what was at stake for those who choose to write, but what was at stake for those who choose to guide people into those hidden places. I returned to the writing warriors I met in my classrooms, the writers who showed me what it takes to be authentic. And I learned that unless I remain a constant student, not just of the craft of writing, but of its process and of myself, I will quickly become a fraud. I will turn into the didactic, rigid writer who speaks more than she listens, who rants more than she questions. I didn't want to be that writer. I didn't want to be that teacher.

I continue to learn something new about writing, the role of writing, and myself as a writer every day. *If I pay attention.* That's the anchor beneath it all. Pay attention. Notice what is, not what I want something to be. I must remember I am always a beginner, always a student, of the art of writing and of life. If I forget that and believe I have mastered something, I inevitably fall on my face and have to start again.

Throughout the book I will talk about the importance of letting something go. When I bring this up in workshops, students often ask questions such as:

- Do you mean something emotional or spiritual?
  Or something physical?
- What does this have to do with writing?
- Do you really mean every day?

Here are the answers:

- Yes, yes, and yes.

- Everything.
- Yes.

And here's why:

We don't write in a vacuum. Our work comes from us, and we inhabit a space. The most intimate level of that space is our body. The next level is the house where our body lives. Then our neighborhood. Our town. Our state. And on and on. If we purge something from our homes, we'll likely notice that we've purged something on an emotional or spiritual level. For example, the tightness over the loss of a lover may vanish when your last pictures of him or her find their way out of your home. Conversely, doing emotional and spiritual clearing will frequently result in a cleansing of our physical space as well.

Let it go. Don't overidentify with either material things or emotional matters. And don't classify one type of healing as more valuable than the next. Donating a pair of shoes to Goodwill is no more or less valuable than doing personal grief work. Resist the temptation to operate from a place of dualism, to say, *This matters; this does not.*

Let it go. Cluttered writing is writing that is simply carrying too much. It's overladen with adverbs or adjectives. It restates itself over and over again. It tries to tack on too many phrases to modify a noun or verb. This leaves the reader hacking her way through your brambles to find out what you meant to say. Pare down your work. You don't have to develop a minimalist style like Hemingway if that doesn't feel natural for you. Find the simplest, most concise way to say what you want to say in the way that you need to say it. This style will be different for every writer. Just check every word. What is it doing? Is it serving the sentence? The paragraph? The chapter? How? If you can't figure out how, cut it. If you notice five words doing the same thing, cut four of them.

When you let go of what is no longer necessary, the authentic essence of yourself and your writing bubbles up. This is freedom. This is flexibility. This is being utterly, completely alive. Are you ready? Take a deep inhale. Expand your belly. Now, let it all go. Hold nothing back. Relax your jaw. Release your shoulders. Soften your gaze, and step into yourself, one warrior word at a time.

## PART ONE

# Breaking Ground

CHAPTER 1

# The Way of the Writing Warrior

If true freedom is going to survive within you, you
have to be willing to fight for it. You have to have a
sword in each hand at all times. One sword is for
your own mind and the other sword is for everyone
else's mind. You must be ready to use them. Anyone who wants to be truly free must be willing to
stand alone in the truth.

—Andrew Cohen

The beginning always starts off easy. "I want to write
a book," you say. So maybe you take a class or two.
Maybe you buy a book on writing. Maybe you join
a critique group. In the beginning, you are filled with possibilities, burning with potential and promise. In the beginning, you really believe that in one semester you can learn
all there is to learn about writing and be on your way to the
Great American Novel. And then the beginning, a time of
sweet kisses and daily flower deliveries, turns into the middle. Ideas that were once svelte and flexible and able to party

until three o'clock in the morning turn into the same old stories, the same old conversation over and over.

"This is no longer love!" you exclaim, and toss your idea, once burning with fire and promise, onto the pyre of self-loathing and vow to start anew with something fresher, more exciting, more flexible and inspiring than ever before. This new idea's kisses are even sweeter, the flowers more fragrant. *This is the one.* And then this beginning becomes another middle. And this middle has a spare tire around its belly. And this middle lost its job. And this middle's eyesight is failing. What to do? This one was *the one!* Obviously, you don't know how to pick 'em. Next time you'll pick one even younger. Stronger. With a faster car.

Stop.

Anyone can fall in love. Not just anyone can stay in love.

The Writing Warrior's path is about staying in love. The Writing Warrior's path is about ruthless self-study. The Writing Warrior gazes in the mirror and notices, without judgment, what she sees. She is also aware that she cannot see it all. The Writing Warrior acknowledges that he sees the world through lenses, and he knows each lens creates a distortion. He has the courage to remove the lenses as he becomes aware of them, and he also has the courage to know when he still needs a lens.

The Writing Warrior stands steady in the center of her work, not reaching too far into the past or too far into the future. She is rooted to the earth, and her spine reaches toward heaven. She identifies and acknowledges the distractions and illusions in her path and, with compassion and clarity, strikes them down. She is aware of her patterns and any tendencies to get in her own way, and she can laugh at herself, openly and with wide lips.

The Writing Warrior knows his time on earth is finite and wants to live it fully. He knows he has essays to write, stories to share, poems to create, and he knows it is his charge to write them. She knows that writing is sacred, that it carries great power, and that it takes work. She knows that though the stories and poems appear as gifts, they require her diligence, her patience, and her discipline to realize their full potential. He must be alert. She must be faithful.

The Writing Warrior's pen is a sword, used both to slice away the mind's illusions and the illusions of the world around her. The Writing Warrior does not pick up the pen lightly. He respects its power, its magic, and its teachings. He knows it carries responsibilities. She steps up to the page, the morning's battlefield, bows to the pen, the page, and to herself. She is ready to cut away what does not serve. He is ready to carve out a new landscape. The pen is also ready, and bows to the warrior, offering its ink as a sacred covenant.

Welcome to the path. We have been waiting for you.

## CHAPTER 2

# Structure Is Alive

No smallest atom of our moral, mental, or physical structure can stand still a year. It grows—it must grow; nothing can prevent it.

—Mark Twain

S tructure is alive.

Write this down. Keep it in your heart. Move it into your body. Structure is fluid. It's essential, but it must breathe. There must be space around any structure you impose—whether it's around your writing discipline and practice or around the form and shape of an actual project. You must allow air in to the framework you erect. You must allow for some bending, some stretching.

The next chapter will outline the primary practice for this book. It consists of three parts: breathing, shaking, and writing. I offer this discipline as a gift, not a prison. Each section closes with additional writing exercises to help you with your inner writing journey and your primary writing projects. Take what is valuable to you and let the rest go.

Any structure that does not come organically from the person working within it will not hold. Any structure for a novel that does not come organically from the spirit of the work itself will not hold. So proceed deeper into this book with caution. It's likely you'll resist some of the practice structures I suggest. That's OK. But it doesn't mean you shouldn't try them. It also doesn't mean you should do them forever. Anything that doesn't have fluidity will freeze, and being frozen is the last thing you want—in your writing or in your body. Throughout the book I will remind you to look within and ask yourself what is authentically right for you. You, not me, must have the discerning eye for your practice. Are you choosing not to do something because it isn't the right thing for you, or are you choosing not to do something because you're practicing avoidance? Only you will know the truth.

I have provided a sample structure because structure is essential. However, just like with clothing (no matter what the labels say), a one-size structure does not fit all writers. There are many paths to the same center. But most writers I've worked with, myself included, need someplace to start.

The breathing practice I ask you to begin with helps you quiet down and settle into your body and your space.

The shaking practice brings you quickly into your body and, since the body is a holistic organism, as you move energy through it, you will break up stagnation and make space in your mind. (Don't be scared! I'll explain this later.) Remember, the mind is indeed a part of the body, not its own separate entity—much though it would like to be! Making space within allows our art to flow. The shaking practice is simple and fast; however, there are many ways into the body. Try shaking. If it's not a fit, then dance, jog, practice yoga, qigong, or gymnastics; find a physical outlet that creates opening, not contraction, for you. But don't be afraid of the shaking just because it's unfamiliar.

And finally, the writing practice should be obvious in its intent—thou must write! But it's more than that. Because of the order of the practices, the writing will often serve more to stretch your writing muscles than to develop a character study or dramatic scene. It's not the content of the writing that matters here. It's the consistency. Just like you can't run a marathon well without training and stretching, you can't expect to show up at your writing area without priming the pump with some consistency. That's what we're looking for with the writing practice—consistency regardless of the outcome. This will help you recognize that your writing, like your body, is different every day. You are not a machine. You cannot produce the same number of pages or words every day for the rest of your life.

You cannot do the same thing every day and remain in balance. Don't create a structure that does not honor your humanness. After all, it's your humanity that allows you to see that dogwood tree in just that perfect way so you can write a haiku. It's your humanity that allows you to experience the wide range of emotions that will allow you to create a compelling plot. It's your humanity that makes you just like all the rest of us and uniquely you. Honor it. Don't fight it.

Structure must have flexibility. Don't be afraid to play with the edges of the structure provided here. Allow it to change as you change. Don't feel like you have to do this every day forever. Listen within. Go within. The structure that you need will emerge, and it will have more staying power because it came authentically from you. Use the structure in this book as a foundation to leap into what only you can create.

Resist the urge to look for a single Holy Grail guide for your writing practice. You are not the same person each day. When you find a practice that works, commit to it, but be flexible with that commitment. The time may come when it is no longer a fit, and you may feel that you've "failed" at your writing practice. Don't place the blame outward. Instead, reflect inward. What didn't work for you and why? Be honest. What would you rather do? Or are you observing simple laziness?

Allow for this freedom in your writing too. Yes, you need a container. That container may be a scene or a character or a driving question. But let there be room to bounce around within the container. Don't hold too tightly to an outcome or a result. That may keep your characters marching in line, but it won't let them speak with their own voices. As a writer, be ever respectful of your characters' voices. Let them know that you are there and that you will love them no matter what they say.

Though the bones of a human body create a person's frame, they are not the person. For there to be life, there must be air—breath and the space within the vertebrae, space within and around the organs. For there to be life, there must be water—the fluids of blood, saliva, water. For there to be life, there must be fire—the electricity of the heart's pulse. And for there to be life, there must be earth—the flesh itself, the ivory of the teeth, the eternity of the bones. You can arrange a skeleton's structure, but you won't get a human being. For that, you need that bit of magic that occurs when everything is in perfect order. And for that to occur, you need patience and persistence.

Show up. That's all anyone can ask of you, and indeed, that is all you can do. Show up. No conditions. No preconceptions. No agenda. See how light that feels already? Conditions, preconceptions, and agendas are bulky and heavy. There's no need to clutter up your writer's self with any of that baggage. Lose it on the connecting flight, sit back, and relax. It's not as complicated as you think.

CHAPTER 3

# The Practice

Be regular and ordinary in your life, so that you
may be violent and original in your work.

—Gustave Flaubert

The foundation for your Writing Warrior path is a
three-part practice. It consists of a three-part breathing exercise, a shaking practice, and a writing practice. Please do this practice for a minimum of forty-nine
days, no matter how far along you are with the writing exercises in the book. Forty-nine days allows you to practice commitment. It is long enough for you to see the effects on your
body and your writing. It is long enough for you to experience any discomforts that arise and bear witness to the wide
range of avoidance tactics you may find yourself using. These
observations, without judgment, are key to your understanding yourself as a writer.

The practice can be done in fifteen minutes if that's all
the time you have. On days you have more time, stretch the
practice out for an hour or longer. The most important aspect
is consistency. Give yourself the gift of discipline. We're all
human and our lives are not the same every day, so don't
beat yourself up and walk away from the whole thing if you

have to miss a day's practice. Just begin again. You're learning to build a relationship with these exercises, the strength of which will carry over into your relationship with your writing. This practice will help to center and ground you and will help you develop intuitive listening and compassion. Please do the exercises in the order presented. Have pen and paper handy for the last part of the practice.

A few things to remember:
- You are not trying to get anywhere or achieve anything.
- You are not trying to look like a yogi or write like your most beloved author.
- You are not going to feel the same today as you are tomorrow.
- You are not always going to want to do this practice. Do it anyway.

## THREE-PART BREATHING PRACTICE

Three-part breathing is fundamental to the Writing Warrior's path. It will also help train you to breathe properly throughout your day. Don't worry if it feels weird. Many of us don't breathe properly. We tend to breathe shallowly into the chest rather than deeply into the belly, and we rarely completely exhale. Three-part breathing will help bring awareness to your breath, as well as fill your body with more oxygen. You may do this standing, sitting in a chair, or sitting on the floor. If you sit in a chair, keep both feet rooted flat on the floor. If you are sitting on the floor, prop enough blankets or pillows under your hips so that your hips are higher than your knees. (Sit on the front edge of the blanket, and let your knees relax down toward the floor.)

Begin by placing your hands on your navel and press firmly. Take a deep inhale and fill your belly, letting it push your hands out and away from your body. Hold the breath for a few seconds. As you exhale, press your hands into your belly as the air releases from your body. Don't be afraid to press your palms into your belly; you won't hurt anything. This will help to promote diaphragmatic breathing. Many people pull their bellies in on an inhale rather than pushing their bellies out. This forces the air up into the chest, resulting in shallow breathing. We want to move that breath into the belly. Continue breathing like this for at least one minute until you can feel your breath pumping slowly into your abdominal region.

When you feel like you've mastered the rhythm, expanding your belly on the inhale and collapsing your belly on the exhale, move your hands up to the bottom of your lower ribs. With four fingers of each hand in front wrapped around the lower ribs, point your thumbs toward your back. Inhale and press your ribs out. Exhale and push your ribs in. You're actually doing this movement with your breath, not with your hands. Your hands are there to help you bring awareness to your rib cage. The ribs can actually expand and get wider with each inhale, and contract on each exhale. This helps to increase your lung capacity. Stay with this movement for at least one minute.

Then take your fingers and place them over your clavicles, also known as your collarbone (the top bone of your shoulder on your front). This is where the last bit of breath fills your body. First the breath goes to your belly, then to your lungs, and then up to your clavicle area. Breathe deeply; feel the breath fill your belly, expanding it, then rising to your ribs, expanding them out wide, then lifting your clavicles as you finish the last bit of inhale. When the breath reaches the clavicle area, the clavicles will lift up, expanding the rib cage even further. Then release and slowly breathe out from your clavicles, past your ribs, and emptying your belly. Think of your body as a vessel. When you pour water into the vessel, the water is first going to fill the belly, then the lungs, and then finish at the top of the chest.

As you practice this breathing, think of expanding your belly and your ribs in four directions: front, back, left side, right side. Once you feel comfortable with belly breathing and full body breathing, you can relax your hands, letting them rest in your lap in a comfortable position, and enjoy the experience.

*Minimum time: five minutes.*

## SHAKING PRACTICE

The shaking practice is the second part of our foundation practice. It's just like it sounds. We're going to shake our bodies. I already hear your resistance through the ether! What's this shaking thing? What does that have to do with writing? I don't understand it. How do I do it right? What's the point?

Most people have been introduced to deep breathing at some point in their lives, and, of course, the idea of a timed writing practice is nothing new either. But shaking? Yeah, I know. It's weird. I thought so too. When I teach it in workshops and classes, the students generally think so too. Until they try it for a while and then send me e-mails telling me how well it worked.

The shaking practice is not complicated or esoteric. Dogs shake when they get out of the bath. We spontaneously shake out our wrists or ankles when they are stiff. Dancing is a form of shaking. A mindful shaking practice will have transformative effects on the practitioner. As writers, when we break up the stagnation within our body, we open up energy channels, enabling us to sink quickly into a more profound and authentic relationship with our writing.

This may seem too easy, or just plain strange. When I first learned the shaking practice, I hated it. It made me itch and it made me cranky. But I was told to shake daily for ninety days as part of my round of Taoist yoga training. I trusted my teacher, so I shook. After a few days, the shaking became less annoying. Then it became fun. Then I began to notice an unexpected lightness. I began to notice more energy and a more immediate connection to my writing—to the writing I was currently engaged with and to new stories floating on the horizon. Shaking helped me be more present. It helped me let go of what I didn't need, and it created space for what needed to move in. I had not expected this.

I began to teach shaking in my writing classes, and I discovered that my observation was not a fluke. Students opened up quickly (after the requisite period of whining). Their writing became much more present and direct. They couldn't hang out in intellectual abstractions. The shaking allowed them to fully embody their skins, which allowed them to fully embody their writing. They learned to be present with what they were feeling and to let it go when the feeling was complete. In order to write authentically, we must know how to go into darkness and we must know how to return cleanly. Shaking helps us cultivate this. It allows things to surface naturally and fall away naturally.

Here's the best thing about the shaking practice: You don't have to set an intention for it. You don't have to know what you want to work through. You don't have to create a framework for it to reveal its secrets to you. You just have to show up and shake and then observe yourself over the days and weeks that you're shaking. Shaking without an agenda, breathing without an agenda, and free writing without an agenda will help teach you to detach from an outcome. It will help free you from limitations in your work you may not be aware of. Shaking isn't about knowing anything. It's about not knowing. There is no wrong way to shake. It's the body's normal response to help eliminate stiffness and stagnation.

## How to Shake

Begin by standing with your feet together, knees soft, jawbone relaxed, tailbone slightly tucked, and your tongue lightly touching the roof of your mouth behind the tooth ridge. On an inhale, step your right foot out to the side and set it down. You're now in a wide-legged stance. Exhale. On the next inhale, raise your arms above your head while rising up on your toes if possible. Hold your breath and sink into a squat, coming only as low as is comfortable. If squatting is not possible, then simply skip the squat, lower your arms on an exhale, and begin to shake. If you do move into the squat, when you're ready, exhale and leap up from the squat, landing solidly with both feet on the floor, and begin shaking. You do not have to jump. You can keep your feet rooted to the ground the entire time. The shaking originates from within your belly. It can be soft and internal, or it can be more energetic and external. Each day your body will tell you what it needs.

The first few times, you may want to pretend you're being shaken by something else just to get your body moving. Don't worry about what you look like. Nobody is watching. Once you get the hang of the movement, begin to focus on your belly in the place between your navel and pubic bone. Let your shaking originate from there. That center of our bodies is our place of power and stability. Imagine a red or orange ball of light in your belly. This helps bring heat into your belly and starts generating internal movement.

There are lots of options available to you now. You might like to pretend that you're really cold and shiver. You might feel energetic and want to jump a bit. You might want to keep your eyes closed, or only slightly open. Try not to let your eyes wander around the room, though. You're allowing energy to disperse through your eyes when you do that.

During the shaking practice, allow your mind to travel through your body, sending energy and awareness to your eyes, ears, nose, throat, teeth, tongue, shoulders, back, spine, elbows, wrists, fingers, heart, lungs, liver, kidneys, belly, hips, knees, ankles, and feet. You might like to click your teeth together and see how that feels. With loose fists, you might like to tap down the sides of your arms and legs or over your skull. Experiment with all the ways you can get in touch with your body. Linger any place you feel tightness or resistance. Allow your breath to move into those areas and loosen them up. Remember, where your attention goes, energy goes, so use this opportunity to listen to your body's wisdom and open up to a more intimate connection with your internal body.

Some days you may feel like more vigorous shaking. Some days you may wish to do gentle shaking. The important thing is just to shake. Some days you write for hours and other days only for a few moments. Shaking practice helps this normal flow of things feel more natural and familiar. Remember that you are bringing energy (using attention and movement) throughout your body. You're waking yourself up from the inside out and developing focus and clarity within your mind. Think of shaking as an internal cleansing bath for your body.

You may itch at first. You may feel silly. You may feel tingling in your arms and fingers. These sensations are perfect. Pay attention to your own body and its needs. Some days I am active in my shaking, while other days I keep my feet rooted and do more of an internal shaking.

Each day, when you feel like you've moved energetically through your entire inner body, begin to slow the shaking down until you reach stillness, with your feet firmly rooted on the floor, your arms relaxed at your sides. Bring your feet back together and feel the sensations of your body as it transitions from movement to stillness. When your heart rate has returned to normal, practice the three-part breath once again for a few deep inhales and exhales.

*Minimum time: five minutes.*

## WRITING PRACTICE

Please do this writing practice longhand if you are physically able to do so. As with the three-part breathing and the shaking, we're not trying to accomplish anything in particular with this writing practice. You should be relaxed after the first two parts of the practice. Now just sit down and start writing. Don't worry if you write nonsense. Don't get attached to it if you write something brilliant. Just write whatever is emerging for you. Don't stop to think about it or edit it. Don't worry about whether or not you can "use" it for anything later. We are simply observing our writing in connection with our breathing and our inner listening.

*Minimum time: five minutes.*

Remember: reading about something is not the same as doing it. Observe yourself in all your excitement about and resistance to these concepts. Let your rational mind take a break, and let your feeling self find a way through the merging of body, breath, and language. Show up without attachment. Breathe. Shake. Write. Notice. You are cultivating powerful tools for your Writing Warrior path.

# THE WRITING WARRIOR PRACTICE

Seek freedom and become captive of your desires.
Seek discipline and find your liberty.

—Frank Herbert

At the end of each section you'll find Writing Warrior Practice exercises. These sections provide a summary of the key concepts of the previous chapters and writing exercises in two categories: Internal Conversations, for deepening your relationship with yourself, and Write Now, for deepening your works in progress. You may wish to keep a journal specifically for working through the exercises in the text.

Part 1, Breaking Ground, introduced you to the concept of being a Writing Warrior. I encouraged you to recognize that structure is necessary, but fluid, and I gave you the foundation practices for this book: a three-part breathing practice, a shaking practice, and a writing practice. The foundation practices will introduce you to the concepts of self-observation without judgment, attachment and aversion, and self-study, which will be addressed later in the text.

## INTERNAL CONVERSATIONS

*You can use the internal conversations exercises for personal work. The deeper your relationship with yourself, the deeper your writing becomes. Feel free to use prose or poetry to respond.*

Free write around the words "structure" and "discipline." After a few minutes, stop and look honestly at your responses. What were your connotations and inferences? What made you uncomfortable? Look for the place that is both flexible and strong, the balance between creating a prison cell for your writing or being a limp noodle in your practice.

What resistances, if any, are surfacing for you around the Writing Warrior practice? Are there any fears? Try to find the underlying reason for these resistances. Go deeper than "I don't want to." Listen softly. Pay careful attention to the word choices you use. The words themselves will provide an insight.

What kind of writing practice are you currently engaged in? What about it is working? What is not? Are you willing to adjust your current schedule as you learn more about yourself and your tendencies?

How would you describe your current relationship to your body? Come up with some images that represent that relationship. Do you feel that you deeply listen to the wisdom of your body? If not, are you willing to entertain the idea that you could?

Mentally travel through your body from the top of your head to the bottoms of your feet. Take your time. Along the way, notice any aches, twinges, tightness, or resistances. Just notice. Are there places in your body that you can't see with your internal eyes? (For example, are you able to energetically acknowledge your liver? Spleen? Baby toe?) Just notice. Write a letter of introduction to your body, paying special attention to the parts you have difficulty accessing.

---

## WRITE NOW

*The following exercises can be applied to works in progress or used as prewriting. Feel free to use poetry or prose to respond.*

Take a scene from a work in progress and add the element of a disciplined practice to it. What activity can the primary character engage in in a more disciplined way? For example, could your protagonist take up a daily walking practice? What would change in the scene? What would remain the same? How does it feel to write about a discipline?

Write a scene or poem in which there are no boundaries for the characters or content. There are no rules of physics or laws. Your characters can do anything. What happens?

Write a scene or poem in which a character's physical structure (body) is changing in some way (for example, through aging, illness, a bone break, or sunburn).

Write from the point of view of a character whose physical body is dramatically different from yours (gender, age, height, weight, health). Embody that character's flesh. Engage the character in physical activity (such as running, walking, swimming, or biking). Slow down as you write and really experience each breath, each step, this character takes.

Write a scene of approximately five hundred words using the following rules:

- Every second sentence begins with the letter *n*.
- A cat figures prominently in the first three sentences.

- A character takes a train somewhere he or she is afraid to go.
- A miscommunication creates more trouble.

What happened? How did it feel to write this way? What worked? What didn't?

PART TWO

# *Building Your Foundation*

CHAPTER 4

# Release All Desire
# for Results

He who stands on tiptoe
doesn't stand firm.
He who rushes ahead
doesn't go far.
He who tries to shine
dims his own light.
He who defines himself
can't know who he really is.
He who has power over others
can't empower himself.
He who clings to his work
will create nothing that endures.

—*Tao Te Ching*, chapter 24

The Bhagavad Gita tells us, "The awakened sages call a person wise when all his undertakings are free from anxiety about results." If you're at all like me, the idea of releasing any desire for results causes a visceral response. If I don't worry about where I'm supposed to end up, how will I know when I get there? How will I know if I've achieved what I wanted to achieve? How will I know if I've done anything at all?

I was first introduced to the concept of releasing attachment to results in yoga class. I didn't really buy it then. I did want to be more flexible. I did want to lose weight. I did want to look like someone on the cover of *Yoga Journal.* It didn't take too many months for me to see that the desire for the goal was creating contraction and suffering and preventing me from enjoying the direct experience of the class. My *wanting* got in the way of my *experiencing*.

The first step of building your foundation for the Writing Warrior path is to release any desire for results. This is not the cop out it may sound like. Paradoxically, this letting go allows you to do more, experience more, and create more than you will if you are fixed on a specific end result. It can be very difficult to see the gifts scattered along the sidewalk if your gaze is firmly focused on a destination point. Releasing desire for results allows you to be open and more accepting of what you find along the way. You will not be as quick to discard things just because they don't fit your planned outcome. And often, what you do end up with is far more wondrous than you could have imagined for yourself.

We live in a results-oriented culture. It is natural to impose this way of thinking on our writing. It may feel absolutely ridiculous to try to write without knowing where you're going to end up. That feeling is OK. Pay attention to what your mind is doing. Are you afraid that you're not learning everything possible? Are you comparing your direct experience to an experience of the past, or an expected experience of the future? Are you worrying about getting everything you're supposed to get from the information? Are you questioning your desire to write? Are you wondering when something's going to happen? Where these exercises will take you?

There's nowhere to go. That's the most confounding, frustrating, counterintuitive concept in this whole writing life. There's nowhere to go. Just show up and let everything go. When we stop worrying about whether or not our writing is living up to the goals we've set in our minds, we can enjoy the experience of writing and, in turn, give our writing the space to live and breathe and develop.

Don't write with an agenda. Don't write with a need to accomplish something. Just show up and write. Don't try to make meaning of your writing afterward, but likewise, don't try *not* to make meaning of it. Be in the experience and let everything wrapped up around that experience (what it should be/could be/shouldn't be/might be) fall away. You'll be quite surprised by how far you can go without all that weight holding you down.

## CHAPTER 5

# Direct Experience

You can't have a genuine experience of language except in language.

—Carole Maso

I worked for a time through the Arizona Artists Roster as a writer-in-residence for grade schools and middle schools. One Friday afternoon in late August, I sat at a too-low table in a too-short chair with four Language Arts teachers at a local grade school. I was scheduled to be their writer-in-residence for the month of October, and we were meeting to discuss what I would be covering in their third, fourth, and fifth grade classes. This was my first residency, created more out of financial need on my part than desire to spread the joys of writing to small children, but I was excited and I wanted to do a good job. The money for one four-week residency was five times better than teaching one adjunct creative writing class at the local community college. Even I could do that math. We were waiting on one of the teachers who was still outside on bus duty. These teachers were sweet people. I could see their passion for children and how much they wanted to provide a good experience for their students. One teacher, a petite, bird-like woman with funky red reading glasses opened up her folder and asked, "What approaches are you going to use for the Six Traits of Writing?"

The other polite teachers waited for my answer, as if I'd just been asked something as simple as whether I wanted cream or sugar with my coffee. I felt the scrambling in my brain as I searched for that answer. But the overriding question in my head was: *what the heck are the Six Traits of Writing?* I had a BA in English and creative writing and an MFA in fiction writing. I'd been teaching community college creative writing classes for several years, and I'd already had two books published. I had absolutely no idea what the Six Traits of Writing were. Apparently, I didn't get that memo. Oh my gosh, what did third graders know about writing that I didn't? This was clearly not going to be as smooth as I'd anticipated.

Because these women were sweet, or perhaps because they were used to dealing with long silences following their questions, the red-eyeglassed woman quickly produced a handout in 36-point font. OK, great. Now I'd be able to answer her questions. I had no doubt whatsoever that I was capable of teaching writing. There must be some new buzzwords flying about.

The handout only made it worse.

6 TRAITS + 1

Idea/Content

Organization

Word Choice

Sentence Fluency

Voice

Conventions

Presentation

"These traits are the qualities of writing," said the eye-glassed one.

Really? Uh oh. I hadn't thought I'd be found out so quickly. I knew in my heart of hearts that I'd somehow skated through graduate school with people much more talented than I, and that I'd scammed my way into a teaching position because I have excellent people skills. But I always thought I'd be undone by the PhD sitting in my creative writing class, proving once and for all to me and the whole class that I actually hadn't ever read a single one of Hemingway's books all the way through. Instead, I was going to be defrocked by the third graders of Phoenix, Arizona.

Whenever content fails me, I fall back on people skills. "Well, I thought we'd spend time actually writing."

They nodded in unison. I wanted to cross my legs, but it was impossible in the child-sized chairs. I kept going.

"I thought if we wrote and then talked about what we wrote, it'd be fun. And educational," I added quickly.

One of the women made notes in perfect script.

"Can you give us a list of your activities and how they connect to the Arizona State Language Arts Standards?"

The what? What happened to the writing part? "Sure. I'll e-mail it tonight."

They seemed momentarily satisfied. The bird-like woman held suspicions, I could tell, but she kept quiet. No doubt something in her background had taught her that artists were somehow different and should be given a wide berth before drastic measures had to be taken.

As we sat together, the mishmash of color in the third grade classroom was comforting. Bright yellow suns against cobalt blue skies. Rainbows. Pictures of funny cats and monkeys. Gold stars. It had been over thirty years since I was in the third grade, but not too much seemed different. Except for this Six Traits thing. That was new. How had I managed to write anything without this essential knowledge?

The meeting concluded well enough. I received my classroom schedule and got a tour of the school (follow the yellow footprints for the third grade hall, the green footprints for the fourth grade hall, and the blue footprints for the fifth grade hall). I couldn't be sure these sweet women weren't wishing they'd picked another artist—maybe the cute one with the long hair who plays drums and makes a lot of noise, then asks the kids to make finger paintings of the drum rhythms—but they'd already given me the check, so we were on for October no matter what.

Once I got home, it didn't take long to find the Arizona State Language Arts Standards online. Finding them, however, did nothing to ease my concern over actually talking about them. Who wrote these things? Who came up with some kind of rubric for what writing is? More important, how is this kind of theoretical discussion even possible, especially with children? It was going to require my most sophisticated sleight of hand to pull off this gig.

I spent an inordinate amount of time worrying about the first day of my residency. I tried to memorize the Six Traits, but they wouldn't stick. I had to keep fighting the urge to sneeze "bull$*&%" in my hand. I was continuously reminded of my favorite Jean Cocteau quote: "An artist cannot speak about his art any more than a plant can discuss horticulture." Was the school system assuming that writing was an external thing? That if you built the skeleton the heart would just move on in?

I tried to remember third grade. I tried to remember how I had been taught to write, but I couldn't come up with anything. We read a lot in school. We memorized poems and parts of stories. We wrote a lot and had to keep journals. I remembered learning about organization and grammar, but grammar was something separate; it was a way of understanding what had been written, but it wasn't *writing*. What had happened? I thought about graduate school. Did we ever have seminars on how to write? None that I could recall. Did we ever come together and agree on what constitutes good writing? No. In fact, we had lively debates over what worked and what didn't in fiction and poetry. The conclusion ultimately being there was no conclusion. Literature has a big tent. Where would Gertrude Stein fall under *conventions* in the Six Traits system? Where would Virginia Woolf fall under *organization* or Don DeLillo under *sentence fluency*? How would Samuel Beckett deal with *ideas and content*?

While I did understand that the Six Traits system helped give the students some vocabulary for discussing writing, and I did understand that the traits, with the notable exception of voice, were all easily marked right or wrong, which made grading papers significantly easier, I also recognized that this attempt to place a rigid container around what makes good writing would create a problem for students later on. Teaching students they can learn how to write by breaking writing down into manageable chunks, to be mastered bit by bit, isn't going to work.

I know this: one cannot dissect something before it's been alive. The same is true with writing. Neither the Six Traits nor any rule-based view of writing take into account what really makes a piece of writing speak. Maybe we can arm our students with comma and semicolon rules, and maybe we can instill a healthy respect for some form of organization, but ultimately, like any warrior worth his or her salt, we know we have to send them out into their own jungles, their own swamps and seas, and see who's capable of bringing back an original catch.

As the old spiritual song says of the lonesome valley, "No one can go there for you." This is true of your work as writers. No one can write for you. No one can share your direct experience of writing. Sure, you can commiserate with fellow writers, but everyone's experience will be different. Each writer navigates her lonesome valley differently. And it's in the valley, not in the dos and don'ts of syntax, where writers get lost. While theory can help you find new ways of looking at problems and activities, and help you think more critically about your own choices and reactions, what matters most is your direct experience: what you feel and hear when you listen inward. Your own feelings and transformations provide the baseline for your practical path.

Pay attention to yourself and to your patterns. Don't let yourself get in your own way. Be vigilant and compassionate. Be in the writing, not around it. Not under it. Not beside it. Be in it. Let the words you're writing and the feelings you're experiencing while writing wrap around you. Please don't trick yourself into believing that reading about writing and thinking about writing is the same as writing. You know in your heart of hearts that isn't true. As a Writing Warrior, your commitment is to the truth—to seeing things as they are, not as you wish them to be. From that place, you will stand in power and authenticity.

## CHAPTER 6

# Theory and Practice

In theory there is no difference between theory and practice. In practice there is.

—Yogi Berra

took piano lessons for five years in North Carolina, from third through seventh grade. I was never any good, but I practiced, metronome pulsing on the mantel. I don't have a natural sense of rhythm, and although I could read the music, I couldn't breathe that invisible spirit into the notes to make them dance. I was competent enough to go to numerous state recitals and place well, and I was determined enough to believe that if I practiced diligently my short stubby fingers would eventually grow long and slender so that I could reach full octaves, even beyond. I loved ragtime music, and I wanted to be able to play a Scott Joplin piece before we moved to Phoenix. But my hands, already twelve years old, had not stretched enough to reach the notes. I could read them, but I couldn't touch them. They mocked me from high above the treble clef.

The point of the lessons, however, was not to become a concert pianist, though that thought had flitted through my mind. The point was to learn to practice. To learn to show up and go toe-to-toe with an instrument, whether that instrument is a golf ball, a piano, or a blank computer screen. Today I can still read music, but I can't play much. The discipline I learned, however, anchored itself in my bones.

I remember getting frustrated with my piano teacher, Mrs. Leggett, because all we seemed to do was practice. We never *got anywhere.* We practiced scales for fifteen minutes before the "real" lesson began. We worked on "pieces" not songs. I wanted what I still want—to jump through the experience to the culminating event. Knowing life doesn't work that way doesn't stop me from wanting it to.

There is no magic moment when practice becomes perfection. A doctor still practices medicine. A professional athlete still practices his game, even in the playoffs. We writers practice our craft, whether we are writing in our journal, writing a proposal, a novel, or a poem. We lay words one after another in various ways, for various reasons, and each path will teach us something. Your craft is not limited to your genre. Let everything you write be a meditation with words, a game, a puzzle. What would happen if you switched the order of the first and second words in your closing sentence? What would happen if you decided to make that statement a question? What would happen if you began every line with the letter *r*? It's both play and the most serious work of your career.

There really is freedom in discipline. Discipline gives you the container to return home to. Discipline picks you back up when your proposal is rejected. Discipline carries you through when your mother is dying, or your world is too full of turmoil to face. Discipline walks with you and pushes you forward. Without it, you are a kite without a string, pulled east, west, north, south, depending on the breeze of the day. Without it, you are unmoored.

Having a writing practice is critical to your journey as a writer. It's essential to have a habit, a routine, a familiar place to settle in to. Developing a routine in any area of your life makes it easier to have a routine in other areas. A mind and body accustomed to a disciplined practice (and I don't mean you have to get up at four in the morning, forgo all human contact, and give up gluten products) will begin to naturally move toward a place of greater focus and discipline at all times. For writers, having a disciplined writing practice will be especially helpful in eliminating the frustration that occurs when you try to take an undisciplined mind, set it down in front of a computer, and say, "Write! Today's writing day!" The undisciplined mind says, "Yeah right. Look over there at that shiny thing. Look there! No there! Are you hungry? I'm hungry. Let's go to the bathroom. Let's check e-mail." And when you walk away from your writing space in disgust, with yourself and with writing, claiming, "I can't write!" you're telling yourself a lie. You're limiting yourself because of a lack of understanding about how your mind works, and then you let that limitation dictate the terms of future events.

All writers do battle with their minds at some point. All writers must find a way to coexist with their minds. The mind is just a part of your body, like your heart or liver. It's your mind's job to make thoughts, so it does. Don't overidentify with them any more than you'd overidentify with the sound of your breath. Thoughts come and thoughts go. You won't succeed in making your mind stop making thoughts, but you can slow them down. You can release attachments to them. You can use breath work and movement to help calm your mind. But you won't get it to shut up all together. And really, you don't want that. That's dead.

Writers in particular need to be disciplined in their practice because the experience of writing can be so intense. A writing practice illuminates our inner thoughts. It can yank out into the open everything the writer has been trying not to look at. And so the writer often walks away. This is normal; writing is hard. Writing holds up a mirror to our demons. It dares us to look at them, dares us further to write about them, and then dares us even further to share them publicly.

A writing practice brings up our limitations. This is a gift, not a problem. The more we know about what we do and why, the more we are able to make authentic decisions. A writing practice shows us our belief systems about ourselves, our family, our world. It shows us where we need to be right and where we feel invisible.

There is no way to avoid practice. Writing begets writing. There is no way to write but to write. There are no tricks, though there are plenty of diversions. Your discipline, your practice and flexibility, make your writing work. However, any structure someone provides for your writing, including the one in this book, or any structure you create yourself, is only as useful as your ability to work freely within it and to stay centered and focused. When a structure of any kind (a relationship, job, religion, writing practice, city) becomes a prison, it's time to move on. Writers often get in the way of their own writing because they think they are supposed to be somewhere other than nestled in the writing. There is nowhere else to be. The structure or concept doesn't make the writing work. The writing makes the writing work.

Writing will not unlock the secret code to fame and fortune. Writing will not bring about world peace. But what writing will do is bring forth your sorrows and joys, your secrets and your lies. It will bring these out, and, once in daylight, they will vanish and you will find you have space in your body, in your mind, and in your heart. And as one writer opens to herself, she brings that changed being into the world and into her contact with others. She has no attachment to whether others change or not, no attachment to whether they write or not; she simply is, and in that "is-ness" she is the stand-alone noun, nothing in the way of all that beauty.

Students of all disciplines have long been resistant to practice. Maybe you are noticing new reasons to avoid practice. Perhaps it's spring and you want to be dancing in fields of flowers. Perhaps it's simple human nature to avoid work. Or perhaps you are not ready to commit to writing. Writing, after all, is serious business. You will likely notice your own resistances surfacing. Stand steady. Shake them loose. Don't be the obstacle on your own path.

CHAPTER 7

# Attachment and Aversion

Attachment is the great fabricator of illusions; reality can be attained only by someone who is detached.

—Simone Weil

You know quite well, deep within you, that there is only a single magic, a single power, a single salvation . . . and that is called loving. Well, then, love your suffering. Do not resist it, do not flee from it. It is your aversion that hurts, nothing else.

—Hermann Hesse

Writers are always finding ways to get in the way of their writing. We grab onto the desire to be published, we become attached to a plot that isn't working, or we become so attached to an image that we squeeze all the life out of it. We avoid doing the very thing we know we need to do—show up, stay put, and write. I know it isn't as easy as "just do it." I know that in order to stay in the chair, you need to face parts of yourself you may have kept hidden for decades. I know it takes courage to tell the truth to yourself and about yourself. Attachment and aversion are the two sisters of suffering. If you're human, you're intimately involved with both of them. They are shadows of each other, and they love to dance on the writer's path.

When I was young, I had a baby blanket that I loved. I slept with it. Carried it around the house. I had planned to take it to school when I started kindergarten, and I remember telling Mom I was going to have it at my wedding. What I loved most about the blanket was its smell. I don't remember that it smelled dirty; it just smelled like me, which likely was dirty if I'd never had the blanket out of my sight for four years.

One day Mom told me she was going to wash the blanket, and she gave me a new blanket to hold. The new blanket wasn't the same as the old blanket. It was thicker, a different shade of white, and it didn't have the fraying ribbon edge that I loved to rub between my fingers. It turned out Mom hadn't planned to wash my blanket. She threw it away and hoped I wouldn't notice. To be fair, Mom and I hadn't known each other long enough for her to know that I noticed everything, but more importantly, she couldn't have known yet that once I loved something, I loved it forever. One blanket can't be replaced with another blanket.

I don't remember how I found out, but I know she ended up getting my blanket back out of the trash. I'm sure there was loud screaming and much stomping of feet. I'm sure she thought it was time I got rid of the baby blanket. I'm sure she was right. But I'm sure of this too: I've still got that blanket in my nightstand.

A baby blanket might be a small thing in the course of a life, but it is a symbol of the larger issues of attachment and aversion. It may be easier to see a toddler's attachment to a baby blanket than an adult's attachment to an unhealthy behavior pattern, but it's the same underlying principle. If a child is attached to her baby blanket, then ask yourself, what is that child avoiding by holding on? Moving into the next phase of life? Putting away childhood things? Losing something familiar?

The answer is an individual one, but the concept is universal. Being attached to something is connected to having an aversion to something else. Perhaps I want to avoid intimacy, so I am attached to a relationship that only partially meets my needs. In the world of writing, perhaps I'm attached to the idea of publication because I'm avoiding a fear of anonymity, a fear of not mattering in the world. Perhaps I'm attached to a particular story arc (which all ten of my closest writer friends have told me doesn't work) because I'm avoiding the issues I'd have to look at if I altered the plot line.

Reverse the idea. What if I avoid sending my work out in the world because it might (will) get rejected? Perhaps in that avoidance, I'm also attached to a faulty idea of what it means to be a writer. Perhaps I avoid sending manuscripts out into the world because they might be accepted. Then, instead of just having a small circle of readers to which I'm attached, more people would read my work, opening me up to criticism. Easier not to send the manuscript out. See how the two ideas are intertwined?

It can be challenging to identify these obstacles in our own writing. Attachments and aversions arise from past experiences. Most frequently, attachments are connected to past experiences of pleasure and aversions are connected to past experiences of pain. But we can take this deeper. Many of us become attached to unhealthy story lines or patterns in our lives because we believe things will always unfold as they did once upon a time. For example, you may refrain from sending a story to an online publication because the editor has rejected your work three times. You may assume that it isn't worth submitting anything because you "know" what the outcome will be.

Over a lifetime, we have catalogued and labeled many future experiences as pleasurable or painful based on what happened or didn't happen in the past. This creates both a closed present life and a life governed by things that already have occurred, not by things that are occurring right now. Attachments and aversions keep us from seeing clearly what is before us to write.

After returning from a trip to North Carolina last year, I wrote a young adult novel feverishly. I hit a wall with it and went to see my teacher. "I'm afraid of getting stuck in these emotions again!" I said. "I have worked so hard to let them go." I feared being unable to move in and out of old feelings as the writing required. I both had an aversion to accessing those emotional areas of my life and felt attached to a past experience that told me I tend to get stuck. Even though the past experience was not pleasurable, the attachment was to the belief that the story line would always play out the same way. Remember, Writing Warriors: The writing does not block us. We are always the ones in its way.

Attachment and aversion in writing are perhaps best observed when you have the gift of finding yourself blocked. When this occurs, rather than stomp away mad, be grateful for the opportunity the block is giving you to learn more about how you get in your own way. Ask yourself: What am I avoiding in this writing? What issues are these characters or this essay or poem working with? Where can I see connections to my own experiences of pleasure or pain? What scares me in this scene? What do I want to have happen? What personal attachment might this writing be connected to? Where there is attachment, there is most likely aversion, and vice versa. As you use the Writing Warrior's sword to cut away these illusions, your path "miraculously" becomes clear. It's not a miracle, though. It is you showing up and doing the work.

In 1977, a year after my dad's heart attack, on summer nights when he felt up to it, he joined the other neighborhood men on their green-and-white plastic Kmart lawn chairs and talked about whatever Southern men in their mid-thirties talked about. My sister and I played kickball with our neighbors, and then tag, running in and out of their house, which was a split-level and so much cooler than our small, single-story ranch house.

We loved the endless stretch of a summer evening and hearing the men's voices, comforting as a summer quilt. Several of the men had a beer in their hands—Schlitz or Pabst— the poor Southern man's nectar and truth serum. Jimmy Carter was president. Nobody liked him but my father, even though he was one of us, a soft-spoken Southern gentleman. It seemed to me that these men sitting together and talking in a North Carolina dusk could fix anything. At the very least, they could fix your car or your riding lawnmower, if not your father's heart.

I loved this time of day because the fireflies were blinking. Slow bugs, they were easy to catch in the palm of my hand. They had a patch of red on their backs, and their light was an ember. They were even easier to catch in a Mason jar. Once, I sealed them in and poked holes in the lid for air, believing that the only thing the bugs needed to survive was oxygen. Of course, in the morning they were dead, even though I'd poked a dozen air holes in the jar lid. I cried because I hadn't meant to kill the bugs; I only wanted to save their light.

I became a writer in part because of my extreme attachment to things. I attempt to capture, preserve, and freeze time. Like catching a firefly, though, it is in the capturing that the death begins. The tendency of many writers, myself included, is to want to freeze the moment, but that's really the antithesis of what needs to happen for a reader to become engaged with a story or idea. The moment must move. You must relax your grip on it so it can expand. The writer's paradox is to hold the moment closely enough with language to give the reader a container to explore it, but not so tightly that the reader suffocates, along with the moment.

A book is not a series of still images; it's a motion picture, an exploration of the constant change of life. The breath and the movement of the breath through your body allows movement to occur on the page. You must not affix too tightly to an image or idea that you want to communicate. You must trust the writing, and you must trust yourself; listen deeply and distinguish between what your ego is writing and what your authentic self is writing. Both attachment and aversion keep us out of direct experience. The farther we are from direct experience, the farther our writing (which by the nature of the craft is a step removed from the experience) will be from the energy of the moment.

A scene's movement engages the reader, not its stagnation. A static scene grants only passive participation. A reader will forget something she passively experiences. He won't so quickly forget a moment he was involved in. Accept the transience of form—of body, of breath. Breath is our transportation from one moment to the next. Your stories float in on the element of air. Dance with them. Feel how light they are when you aren't the one holding them down.

# THE WRITING WARRIOR PRACTICE

No horse gets anywhere until he is harnessed. No
stream or gas drives anything until it is confined.
No Niagara is ever turned into light and power
until it is tunneled. No life ever grows great until it
is focused, dedicated, disciplined.

—Harry Emerson Fosdick

Part 2, Building Your Foundation, introduced you to the
fundamental concepts that will root you on your Writing Warrior path. As you learn to release your desire
for results, you'll find freedom and clarity in your writing. Letting go of expectations teaches detachment and allows you to
be in your direct experience rather than in your past or future
concept of that experience. Deepening your understanding of
the difference between writing theory and practice will help
you move from an intellectual acknowledgment of ideas to a
visceral understanding of experience and its effects on you. As
you become more present in your writing practice, your work
will naturally deepen. You don't need to force it. Being able to
recognize your attachments and aversions will help you avoid
remaining stuck in patterns and beliefs about your writing
that are no longer serving you.

Remember to return to your three-part breathing practice, your shaking practice, and your writing practice. They are your safety practices, your companions, your guardians. They will hold you when you thrash about in the wind. They will give you the freedom to fly because with them, you are firmly grounded.

---

## INTERNAL CONVERSATIONS

*You can use these internal conversation exercises for personal work. The deeper your relationship with yourself, the deeper your writing becomes. Feel free to use poetry or prose to respond.*

Consider keeping a journal just for your reflections and awarenesses around your writing practice. How frequently have you shown up to practice? Don't judge yourself. Just observe.

What have you observed throughout your daily life now that you've incorporated the breathing, shaking, and writing practices?

The shaking practice helps keep impurities (undigested food, disease, and emotional issues) from building up in your blood, tissue, and bones. You may experience some sneezing, coughing, itching, or changes in your elimination schedule. Your body is getting rid of what it doesn't need anymore. What have you noticed?

Take inventory of your space, both internal and external. Look with a discerning, nonjudgmental eye at your inventories. What can you let go of today?

Look honestly at your writing process. Pay careful attention to your writing time, your writing place, even your thoughts and attitudes toward writing. What are your unique resistances to writing? What pulls you to write? Nobody is standing over your shoulder to make sure you write this week. The more you understand your process, the softer your relationship with writing will become.

What are you worried about that you haven't yet experienced? How far into the future are you thinking? No judgment. Just notice.

We truly are a results-oriented culture. What would you do/could you do if the end result didn't matter? Write a letter to yourself. Are there ways you can incorporate these ideas into your life now?

---

## WRITE NOW

*The following exercises can be applied to works in progress or used as prewriting. Feel free to use poetry or prose to respond.*

Place your character in a situation in which he or she is incapable of moving, either physically or psychologically. What happens?

Describe a setting in one of your stories or poems by relating what is not there.

Allow your character to take an inventory of the things in his or her bedroom. What is the character most attached to? Write a scene in which the character must let the item go.

What is your character worrying about? What keeps him or her up at night? What would happen if that thing occurred? Write the scene in which it does.

## PART THREE

# Dissolving Your Illusions

## CHAPTER 8

# The Writer's Wheel of Suffering

Because you're not what I would have you be, I
blind myself to who, in truth, you are.

—Madeleine L'Engle

We're sitting together on metal folding chairs in a lopsided circle. Some of us are smoking cigarettes. Some of us are on our fourth Styrofoam cup of coffee. Some of us have nervous twitches, or the shakes. We're in a moldy basement, or an attic, or a meticulously furnished living room in a swanky suburb. No one wants to begin. We look at each other, or deliberately away from each other. We hold our Styrofoam cups to our lips longer than it takes to swallow a sip of coffee. Finally, a pale man, slightly bowlegged, with dyed black hair and black-framed glasses, speaks.

"Hi. I'm Brian."

"Hi, Brian!" we say.

His gaze scans the room, never landing long enough on anyone to make a connection. His feet shuffle. He opens and closes his mouth, until, at last, "And I'm a writer."

We let out collective breaths and applaud. "Welcome, Brian!" We are jubilant that someone has made the first move. Jubilant that we can all immediately start the comparison game, our minds happy to be free to disconnect once more from the direct experience of the moment and instead, joy of joys, invest in tinkering with someone else. *At least I'm not as bad off as he is. Wow, he's a mess. I'm so together compared to him. Thank goodness he spoke and not me. Is anyone looking at me? Is now a good time to go and get another cup of coffee? Maybe I could step outside now, even though I don't smoke, just so no one will think I could be anything like this guy . . .*

"It's been three days since I last wrote anything. Seven months since I sent anything out. Five years since I published anything."

Now the room is still. We hold our cups midpath to our mouths. We want to look away, but we can't. We're witnessing the train wreck we're all a part of. He's no longer someone "other." He and we are the same, and he's bought into the biggest illusion of all: the Writer's Wheel of Suffering.

The Writer's Wheel of Suffering is that great writer's hamster wheel we've all taken a trip on at some point. It is the wheel that keeps us leaping from one illusion to the next, chasing the invisible carrot that we believe will take our suffering away. All this jumping around makes the wheel spin faster, which causes us to become more afraid of stopping the wheel and, heaven forbid, getting off it. After all, chasing illusions has become so familiar and comfortable we perceive it as reality.

Suffering leads to suffering. Chasing illusions results in an attachment to the chase. Writers love to lament the state of publishing, the hackwork being published, the lack of time to write, the need for more money, more solitude, more companionship. Put a bunch of writers together and, within moments, someone will bring up a reason to be suffering.

Don't buy into this. It may feel real. It may feel like the only choice you have if you embark on the writer's path, but it is not. You can make other choices.

Sometimes I feel as if writing classes should be less about the craft of writing and more like a support group. Craft goes down pretty easily. It's not hard to demonstrate how to make a sentence better or to point out a logic flaw in an idea. The ever-increasing ways in which we can make ourselves suffer—the lengths to which we'll go to ensure that we are suffering—never cease to amaze me. I watch it in myself too. We suffer when we take ourselves out of reality and view ourselves as individuals outside of normal life experiences. "Real" writers don't have a blissful writing experience every moment. Published authors still get rejections. Really good books don't always sell. That's the experience. That's the norm. Don't fight that by thinking your experience should be different.

A student in my class last semester commented that he could tell things to our class that he couldn't tell anyone else, including his wife, because she wasn't a writer. While I don't doubt the sincerity of his comment, and I do see the value in meeting in groups with common interests, I've noticed that writers attach a great deal to the idea of being different from everyone else. Imagine: back of the hand pressed against the forehead, body in a slight swoon, "No one understands me!" Follow it up with a deep sigh, and then look around quickly to see if everyone is paying appropriate homage to the Great Misunderstood Writer.

It's OK to smile a little now. Laugh even. It's OK to admit that you recognize part of this Great Misunderstood Writer within yourself. This writer begins sentences with: "If only I had enough money, I'd . . ." or, "If only I had six months off, I'd . . ." or, "They just publish shlock these days. There's no room for real literature anymore." Or, "Everyone knows those contests are fixed." Or, "I got passed over by this editor because all she wanted was (fill in the blank with your most hated type of book)." Starting to get the picture? Try taking a look at these statements for what they are: ways of not participating in the reality of your direct experience by either attachment or aversion. Direct experience is nonnegotiable, but the stories you make up about it can change, and as they change, you'll find freedom and space.

If you understand that suffering arises when we want our current experience to be something other than what it is, you'll see how much we, and not events, bring about our suffering. Take care not to get caught in the wheel's spokes here. I've seen too many talented writers spin their lives and gifts away by being too attached to a particular outcome or too intent on avoiding something in the writing itself, or in their careers. When this occurs, we are ultimately having a clash with the contents of our minds. Recognize this is an internal issue, and know that you can regain power over the choices you make. If you perceive you are a victim to outside forces, you are sentencing yourself to a lifetime on the wheel.

When I was learning to play piano, my mother told me, "If you don't practice, you'll never get any better." But I never had to be told to go to my room and write. I wrote because writing was the most important thing to me. I thought about writing when I wasn't writing. I thought about what my future as a writer might be. I thought about being the youngest person ever to publish a book (a dream that was dashed quickly when an eight-year-old boy published a book). I thought about being the first female president of the United States and I thought about being a concert pianist, but I knew those two dreams were really just dreams. Not only was I certain writing was possible for me, I knew it was inevitable. I practiced the piano because my mother told me to and because I wanted to play well, but I didn't have a lot of fire for it.

As a child, I couldn't imagine ever not loving every minute of writing. I couldn't imagine the time not being mine to do with as I pleased, or a time when I felt I had nothing to write about. But those times arrived as an adult, and I was caught off guard. I felt betrayed by writing, and I felt that if I couldn't do the only thing I ever wanted to do, then I might as well sell out to Evil Corporate America and make a zillion dollars. I did sell out to Evil Corporate America for a while, but I didn't make a zillion dollars, and, more important, I never lost the pull to write. Not that I always wrote, mind you, but I felt sharply the absence of writing in my life if I didn't practice. I felt guilty when I didn't write, and the longer I stayed away from writing, the more attached I became to my reasons for not writing. The more attached I became to those reasons, the more power those reasons had—not because those reasons were authentic or valid, but because I'd imbued them with the power to alter the way I chose to see my life and the role of writing in my life.

Every semester when I invite my students to introduce themselves and chat a moment about why they're in the class, inevitably someone (often many someones) will say, "I need to take a writing class so I will write." Essentially, they're asking someone else (me) to be their mother—their outside reason for writing, just like my mother was my outside reason for practicing piano. That's OK. I understand that one of my primary roles as a teacher is to provide a structure. We tend to need outside motivation to get started doing something, even, ironically, if it's something we claim to want to do more than anything else. Ultimately, though, each student must find his or her own way, and each student must cultivate the desire to practice from within. Any outside motivation for practice will at some point fall short. A class or two can kick-start you again. A dedicated writer's group can sustain you when you feel like everything you write is garbage. But no one is standing over your bed with a whip or a carrot. There's you and you; best find a way to negotiate that relationship so that you can serve your writing and, subsequently, the rest of the planet. We need more people doing what they're supposed to be doing.

Being able *to write*, not simply to organize or punctuate, arises when you are able to be at ease with the unique games and distractions your own mind is tossing around. Certainly, we're all unique and are going to experience slightly different manifestations of the spokes on the Writer's Wheel of Suffering. I've been paying attention for a lot of years to myself and my students, and I've come up with the following illusions that form the spokes of the Writer's Wheel of Suffering:

Illusion of Time

Illusion of Thoughts

Illusion of What a Writer Is

Illusion of Identification

Illusion of Control

Illusion of Distractions

Illusion of Publication, Success, and Fame

Illusion of Money

Let's take each of these illusions in turn. Our end-of-section exercises will help you look at the roles each one plays in your writing life.

CHAPTER 9

# Illusion of Time

Clocks slay time. Time is dead as long as it is being clicked off by little wheels; only when the clock stops does time come to life.

—William Faulkner

M y grandfather built the house the character Joey lived in on the Warner Brothers' television series *Dawson's Creek*. My grandfather lived on that land in Wilmington, North Carolina, his entire life. He also built the pier, where Joey and Dawson flirted with each other, and he and my uncle rebuilt it after each hurricane that swept through the coastal Carolinas. My father grew up on that land, hunted quail there, picked figs.

When my grandmother died in 1996, my sister and I inherited the cornfield that ran alongside her property and my aunt inherited the house. In 1997, *Dawson's Creek* came to Wilmington and somehow discovered my grandmother's home, which was the perfect location for Joey and *Dawson's Creek*, which is really Masonboro Sound, which is really where we caught crabs every summer in green nets, screaming when they cut loose and scurried across the gray boards of the pier to dive back into the creek. Dad told us an alligator lived there when he was growing up. Sometimes he'd find it when he was swimming in the creek with his sister and his dogs, at least until he contracted polio in 1948 and spent time in an iron lung and then the rest of his time with a right leg shorter than the left, wearing elevated orthopedic shoes to bring him into balance.

My grandmother walked to the pier, where Joey and Dawson had their first kiss, when my father told her we were moving to Arizona. She cried crocodile tears and claimed she'd miss us. Maybe she did. Shortly after my grandmother died, my aunt agreed to lease the house to Warner Brothers for the show, and before we knew it, my father's childhood home was on prime time television.

When my father died in 1987, I was young enough, nineteen, that I would have enjoyed watching *Dawson's Creek* had it been on the air then. When he died, his family did not come to Arizona where we were. They stayed in Wilmington and held a memorial at my grandmother's house, soon to be Joey's house. I always wondered what it was like to hold a memorial service for him without his wife and children. A memorial service for all the people who knew him before he met my mother, before we moved to Arizona—the people who knew him when he could still run, when he was still balanced, left and right, moon and sun.

In *Dawson's Creek*'s fifth season, Dawson's dad died suddenly in a car accident along a stretch of road that my dad knew well. Dawson was nineteen, as I had been, and in his first year away from home at college, also as I had been. A wake was held for his father in Dawson's sprawling Southern house, just across the creek from Joey's house, overlooking the same body of water where my dad had swum with the alligators until he couldn't swim anymore.

Cast members in mourning clothes walked onto the expanse of emerald lawn, a color only found south of the

Mason-Dixon Line. People repressed their grief, ate finger foods, and awkwardly embraced the widow. Dawson's father's ghost hung everywhere. He played with my father's ghost, who I felt clung to the walls as well, though I have come to see that perhaps I affixed him there, in 3-D color, so I would always know where he was.

The fireplace where we had spent so many Christmases was on television—a centerpiece for Dawson's family's mourners to gather, leave teacups and biscuits, and be silently grateful that death hadn't visited them so intimately. The floor where my grandmother had read *Little Black Sambo* to me had been recarpeted a brilliant red for the TV show. But everywhere in the house on the television screen, death hung.

Fifteen years and three thousand miles away, I watched the episode in my air-conditioned living room in Arizona. My body cried out as if it was 1987. As if Dawson's father was my father. As if my grandmother still lived in her house and wasn't many years dead. As if I hadn't spent ten thousand dollars in therapy already. As if time was not linear, but a loop, and Dad was dying over and over and over, equally, every time I rewound the episode. It felt the same, like someone had reached into my belly and pulled out my intestines one foot at a time. It felt the same, whether on TV in 2002 or in my "real" life of 1987. The television program was the play, the dream, the performance, but nothing about its impact was less real than when I had gone home to my apartment alone the first night after Dad died and felt with hurricane intensity that I had to nail him to the wall before I lost him or I would come entirely undone. Was the TV ghost real and my father's ghost the illusion? I have no language for this.

I have tried for years to write about the absurdity of witnessing my grief on TV on a set that isn't a set, but my dead father's childhood house. I hear the monkey of illusion laughing, chattering as I spin in a time warp I've created based on an illusion that time is linear, that it stops and starts and can be contained by a battery and a plastic watch face. An illusion that a story can be contained by a single beginning and a finite end. That the very foundation of my life had been real, or, more accurately, had been more real than anything else I could remember or imagine. Yet the script of *Dawson's Creek* created a bridge that spanned fifteen years to touch emotions in me that had clearly never moved. *Dawson's Creek* showed me in HDTV the absurdity of linear time.

Dawson's dad and my dad can die again any time I pop the tape in. The story is a circle, broken only randomly by my decision to press pause. The story is unattached to my perception of it. It has nothing invested in whether I cry each time I press play. Dawson's dad can be frozen, midcrash, as long as I have the tape stored. He can remain pinned to the wall of the set that isn't a set until my body moves him. I can experience my dad's funeral again, two decades later, because the memory of it never moved. I can be thrown back twenty years in time because of a trigger image on a television screen.

Memory is supposed to be fluid, but often in the throes of trauma, we burn our own DVD of the story. When memory becomes fixed it's no longer true to the nature of memory, which is supple and shifting, choosing details that are pertinent to the current situation. If we solidify a story in our memory, our mind freezes, and the part of our body that carries that memory freezes and we become more rigid and less flexible. As we freeze memory, we freeze time. Only, of course, time cannot stop. Or more accurately, our relationship with time does not stop.

Let me be clear. Time, like your mind, is a tool for your use. An awareness of time ensures that you pay your bills, get to work, show up for your wedding, and remember to vote. An awareness of time helps you manage the things you must juggle in any given day. But time is not a master. Time is an arbitrary ordering of daylight and moonlight. If you ever doubt that, just think about time zones and the international date line. Either it's noon or not, right? Either it's Monday or it's not, right? Think about the towns in the United States where one side of town is on Central Time and one side of town is on Mountain Time. Random. Arbitrary.

Time can appear to stretch or shrink based on your perception of what is occurring. Pleasant events seem to go by more quickly than less-pleasant activities. But the truth is that time just passes. It neither speeds up nor slows down—in no small part because it does not exist. It's a human creation designed to help us better manage our lives. It's as random as calling the sky blue and the grass green. Remember this so you won't be fooled by its perceived importance.

Don't let notions of time determine how successful your writing is. There are no breakout novelists. There are writers who have worked and worked and received rejection letter after rejection letter, and when their first novel appears (which is really the seventh one they've written) they (if they're lucky) get lauded as a "new" talent. They're not new. They've toiled away, day by day, word after word, until something was published. Don't be fooled by the media's need to jump on the newest, fastest, youngest, prettiest thing. It's irrelevant. You write whether you get published or not. You write whether you have a good review, a terrible review, or, perhaps worse, no review at all. You write when it's sunny and when it's cloudy. You write when you're in your twenties, your forties, your eighties—not because you're being showered with financial rewards, but because you're a writer. Let time be the river it is. Let that river carry you from one book to the next. There is no overnight anything.

If you need to think in terms of linear time, then use ten years and ten thousand hours as an average benchmark for a writer before you begin to see some fruit from your labor.

Those ten years are spent not in sitting around a coffee shop talking about being a writer, but in writing, studying, reading, revising, revising, revising. Those ten years are spent accumulating more than a few file drawers of rejection slips, and those ten years are spent having to defend your statement "I am a writer" to people who want to know when your book (which isn't finished or has already been rejected a hundred times) is coming out. Those ten years are spent being a writer. Those ten years can become fifteen years, or they may be only eight years, or for the unusually gifted *and* lucky, just a few years. But don't hang your hat on being a success after your first class or first story publication. Time is neither friend nor foe. Time is a tool. Use it and forget about it.

CHAPTER 10

# Illusion of Thoughts

Attachment is the mind stuck to an object.

—Lama Zopa Rinpoche, *The Door to Satisfaction*

The first house I owned had an evaporative cooler in the kitchen window. It was an old unit, jerry-rigged together on some two-by-fours. A piece of Styrofoam filled in the cracks around the cooler and the window's edge. Dusty blinds covered the other half of the window to keep out the sun. I just assumed the window wouldn't open. After a few years, I decided I wanted more light in the house, so I hired a handyman to come out and measure the glass and order a new windowpane that would open and let in some fresh air. He came over and measured, and then returned with a piece of glass. When he went to install the new glass, he called me over.

"This window opens fine. Did you even try to open it?"

I had to laugh. No. I had never tried. I had just assumed it was shut and stuck. The sunlight had been available to me the entire time.

We find ourselves in dangerous territory when we take our direction from our thoughts, both in our day-to-day lives and in our writing. The terrain becomes even more dangerous when we assume that these thoughts are reality. As Buddha says, "It is our mind which creates this world." In this sense, it's challenging to see the hand of the creator when the creator is you, but you must find a way to begin to notice this. Just as it's hard for us to see our own writing clearly, especially in the initial throes of writing, it's very hard for us to see our own fingerprints on our life's path. What doors have we already closed because we think they can't be opened? What writing ideas have you not allowed yourself to follow because you believe you're not a good enough writer, or the idea has been done too many times before, or you don't think you have anything new to say about it? How many conferences or networking situations have you backed out of because you think you're not good enough yet? How many have you backed out of because you think you're too good? Don't become a prisoner of your thoughts, and likewise don't attempt to master them. They come and they go. They'll always come and go. Let them. When you hang on to a thought, you're breaking the flow of that thought's path. You're keeping it from doing what it is designed to do—arise, pass through, and disappear. Make no mistake; you hold the thought. The thought does not hold you.

It's pretty easy to see how this relationship with thoughts can affect your relationship with your writing, isn't it? After all, when all is said and done, there's just you and you hanging out in that room, or in that coffee shop, or on that mountaintop. If a thought arises that can bully you into quitting, that's a problem. If a thought arises that can convince you that every word that drops from your fingertips is perfect and golden, that's a problem. Thoughts are going to arise. That's what thoughts do. Some days your thoughts are going to be soft and sweet. Other days they may leap out at you with daggers and stab you in the heart.

Don't make thoughts something more than they are. They'll rise to the challenge, and before too long you'll forget they're thoughts and decide they're you. Cut that off at the pass. The practice outlined in the beginning of this book will help you learn to recognize your thoughts for what they are—part of living in these beautiful fleshy bodies. They're just a part, though, not the whole deal. Stay awake and they won't run your life. Fall asleep and you'll find yourself wondering where your life went and who was in charge while you were gone.

## CHAPTER 11

# Illusion of What a Writer Is

Of the first seven novels I wrote, numbers four and five were published. Numbers one, two, three, six, and seven, have never seen the light of day . . . and rightly so.

—Sue Grafton

During the introductions at one of my short-story classes, a beautiful woman with primary-colored jewelry told the class she had enrolled because she was terrified of writing and her advisor had told her she should take a creative writing class to get more comfortable with the writing process. I assured her she was in the right place, and all seemed well. She attended the first three classes, read the assigned reading, and participated in the discussions. Then, on the fourth class, when students were supposed to come with their first writing activity, centered on characterization, she flipped out. She called me, truly afraid of doing the writing. "I don't know how, I don't know how, I don't know how," she kept saying.

I tried to reassure her that if she knew how to do all of it then she probably wouldn't have signed up for the class. I told her to just write something down, anything, and it would be OK. I told her that her mind was getting in her way. I told her to breathe. She came to the class, but she hadn't written anything. She had the opportunity to hear what other students in the class had written, and I told her she could write something for the next exercise. I got another phone call before the next class. "I don't know how to do this. I've never done it before." She was clearly afraid of putting anything down on paper in case it was "wrong."

Nothing I could say could convince her it's never wrong. Writing leads to writing. The crap comes before the good stuff. She held a belief that there are people who are writers and people who aren't, and that those who are writers write daily with great joy and confidence. Those who are writers always know what's going on with their work. They always have something unique to say, and they always use just the right word. They never worry over what they're going to write, and the universe always lauds their work when it (of course) shows up on the best-seller list. Then there's everyone else, the group of which she considered herself a charter member. Everyone else struggles. Suffers. Can't think of anything to say. Writes choppy and sloppy sentences. Writes clichés and melodramatic scenes and stereotypical characters. Everyone else misses the irony in the short story we read that the teacher is going on and on about (real writers, of course, not only saw the irony, but would have written it better, with even more subtlety and finesse).

I encounter this myth about writing and writers enough to give it its own section here. I don't know where it started. Maybe because much of a writer's work is solitary the world at large doesn't see us deleting half our life's work, or pacing our bedroom floors, or staring out the window filled with debilitating self-doubt. The world at large doesn't see the piles of rejection slips—the rejections from graduate schools, from editors and agents, from publishers, from magazines ranging from *The New Yorker* to *Granny's Knitting Quarterly*. These things happen in solitude, so perhaps to the rest of the world, they don't happen at all.

We can look out our windows and see the young boy practicing free throws all day on the weekends. We can stop by the local theatre and watch the hours and hours of rehearsals the actors go through. We can hear the early painful refrains of the young girl learning to play the flute. But our writing that doesn't work is invisible and silent. It doesn't echo through our parents' homes while they're trying to have a conversation. It doesn't create rooms and rooms of failed paintings. Failed writing doesn't take up space at all, except in the writer's psyche; though, if we're paying attention, we know these failed writings are the most valuable of all because each failing taught us something about not just the craft of writing, but about our relationship with writing. Didn't work this time? OK, maybe I'll try it this way. That publication said no? OK, let's revisit the work and then resubmit it someplace else. Those decisions are made alone.

If you are courageous enough to call yourself a writer, the first question out of the stranger-across-the-aisle's mouth will be, "What have you published?" In our society, we're judged on what we've produced, what we've "done." If we dare to call ourselves writers, we may have produced reams and reams of work that hasn't quite worked, but if we haven't sold something, then it's deemed that we've not really done anything at all. This false assumption trickles down into the psyches of hopeful writers and turns us against not only ourselves but against the very process necessary to actually write something that could sell one day.

The effects of this myth are most poignant for me when I encounter a student such as this beautiful woman, who had enough courage to sign up for the class, enough courage to come to class, but then, when faced with what every single writer in the universe is faced with, freaked out and fell into the trap so many people do: believing she's the only one who doesn't have entrance to this secret club of Writers, so she's not worthy of being in their company. She didn't stay in the chair long enough to learn to both do battle with her own mind and see that every other student in the room is facing a similar battle. I beg you: stay in the chair.

Later on in the same class, an older gentleman asked, "Do even good writers revise?" We were two weeks from the end of the semester, and I was practically punch drunk by that point. His question was so innocent and so absurd (though he had no idea it was absurd) that I almost didn't know what to say in response. His question spoke more to the depths of the misunderstandings about writing than anything else.

"Only good writers revise," I said, and was then able to move into a discussion about what revision actually is and that writing a story isn't, contrary to popular belief, like riding a bike. Once you get one down, you haven't in any way assured yourself of getting the next one down, or the next, or the next. Every time you sit in the chair to write, something different occurs. Some new problem, some deeper question about the work or the characters arises. His question spoke so deeply to the self-doubt writers feel when they hold themselves up against the illusion of the Writer. There is no Writer. There is only you and your work. Be proud of the files and files of work you've created that may not have found a home. Nurture the relationship you have with your writing practice and your stories. Don't set your work aside because you can't write the perfect sentence today. Perfect sentences rarely arrive fully formed. They take numerous incarnations to show up on the page in their perfection.

How many hours of practice and broken toes and pulled hamstrings did we not see Baryshnikov endure before his moments of perfection on stage with the New York City

Ballet? He practiced, and fell down, and sweated, and jumped his cue so the moment would come when he didn't fall down or enter the stage too soon. His innate talent and drive pointed him in the direction of practice. Practice gave him the discipline and the stamina to keep dancing whether particular performances were brilliant or not. Practice instilled in him a relationship between dancing and himself that was sacred. Practice provided a foundation for him as he pushed the edges of his art.

Practice will do this for you, too. You must first acquaint yourself with your writing and, perhaps more elusively, with yourself as a writer. You need to find ways of working within the machinations of your own mind, and this will become easier for you as you let go of the Illusion of What a Writer Is. Take this advice from the prolific John Updike: "More than half, maybe as much as two-thirds of my life as a writer is rewriting. I wouldn't say I have a talent that's special. It strikes me that I have an unusual kind of stamina."

No one is drawn to writing for the exact same reason. Some of us are songwriters. Some love the length and breadth of the novel. Still others try to see the world in the rhythm of a poem. Some people want to publish. Some want to leave something of themselves behind for their families. Some want to use writing as a way of deepening their spiritual path or their relationship with themselves, and some enjoy playing with words on a page, seeing what combinations and sounds and meanings they can come up with. No one has cleared your path for you. Don't be fooled into thinking you don't have what it takes. There's no formula for that journey.

Try this: quit writing. Give it up like you'd give up alcohol if you were an alcoholic. Just quit cold turkey and watch yourself. How long can you go before that tug on your soul toward language and stories begins to materialize? How long can you go before the voices and stories that you hear become so loud you can't hear anything else? How long can you keep yourself from doing what is within you to do? Try it. Then write about the experience. What brought you back? What did you miss about it? What is at the root of the pull back to your work? Post these answers somewhere near your writing area so you can return to them and remember why it matters. Remember, also, every writer at some point wonders why it matters. You may need a little help from time to time to remind yourself that it does. You don't have to know why.

A writer opens her heart, even when it is so bloody the exposure to oxygen makes her scream. A writer pries the fingers of the ghosts from her shoulders with the care of a parent. She places them in front of her and looks them in the eye.

"You," she says, pointing to one with a curved back and crossed eyes. "I can work with you today." The ghost smiles, inches closer to her.

"You. I can't work with you now." The dark one with the missing spleen vanishes. She knows it will be back.

"You. Maybe." The red one shakes, afraid to hope.

The ghost with the curved back and crossed eyes strokes the writer's hand.

"What is the first word?" the writer asks.

"Who," says the ghost.

*Who,* the writer writes.

"Am," says the ghost.

*Am,* the writer writes.

"I," says the ghost.

*I.*

The writer exhales, waits, and listens. The ghost with the curved back and crossed eyes waits, inhales, and begins to speak.

## CHAPTER 12

# Illusion of Identification

First, rely on the spirit and meaning of the
   teachings, not on the words;
Second, rely on the teachings, not on the
   personality of the teacher;
Third, rely on real wisdom, not superficial
   interpretation;
And fourth, rely on the essence of your pure
   Wisdom Mind, not on judgmental perceptions.

—The Four Reliances, Buddhist teaching

So, you're a human being. This "being human" thing sure has a pesky nature about it. You're walking along, happily munching on a Balance Bar, focusing on all the things you do well and wondering how you can incorporate more of the things you do well into your life, and then bam! You run headfirst into a tree, nearly choking on your snack. Hopefully, this head-banging is just a gentle tap from the universe, rather than the pull-no-punches wake-up-and-pay-attention thunks that will happen later on if you don't heed the first calls.

What happened? You toppled over because you were out of balance. You placed all your energy into things that come easily for you. You became really strong in certain areas (plot development, maybe, or dialogue construction). You received praise for these things, so you worked on them even more. (And let's be honest, it wasn't that much work; it came easily.) And so while you were tilling the soil of plot development and dialogue, weeds of the thorny variety sprung up in the fields of characterization and sentence structure. And what's the nature of weeds? They spread. They create clutter. They infiltrate. Divide and conquer. Trick you sometimes with pretty yellow or white flowers. The longer you ignore them, the stronger and fiercer they become. The longer you ignore them, the harder it can be to ever venture into those fields again. After all, you've grown so strong in other areas; how could you admit, after all this time, that you've neglected half of your craft? Way too embarrassing. You're way too old to start over. It's way too risky for someone to pull back the proverbial curtain of Oz.

You're going to keep running into trees, though. Eventually, the untended parts of your garden are going to slither across the field and snag you on the ankles. It's human to play to your strengths. But don't give them all your attention. Don't identify with them. Notice what you don't want to do. (Gee, I don't *want* to revise my story! Come on, I don't really need to pay any attention to that plot hole. The ending is so perfect! I don't need to do any research about seventeenth-century Eastern European medical practices, even though my protagonist is a seventeenth-century Eastern European doctor; after all, it's fiction, right?) Fill in your own "but I don't wanna" and laugh at yourself.

You may have heard "the exercise you hate to do is the one you need to do the most" as it relates to physical exercise. The same is true for writing. If you cultivate only those craft components that grow easily for you, you'll quickly be out of sync; even if you write the best dialogue in the universe, your piece won't be balanced. Consciously seek out areas in your artistic development that make you uncomfortable. Don't always read the same types of books from the same types of authors. Don't start all of your stories in the same way. Try writing from the point of view of the opposite gender, or of someone vastly different from you in age or belief system. If you're twenty-five, write from the perspective of an eighty-year-old. If you're a Democrat, see what the world looks like through Republican eyes. Be ever vigilant in challenging yourself to push farther with your craft. It's up to you. No teacher can push you as far as you can push yourself, because only you know your own soul. Only you know when you're hiding in the bushes and avoiding something uncomfortable, or when you're truly out there scrambling for footing. It's in the scrambling that you're most open to the work. It's in the moments when you sway from side to side—when you're not sure, when you don't know—that your work has a microsecond to sneak in and surprise you.

As soon as you begin identifying with a certain element of your writing, you start losing your capacity to see it clearly. It's a common trap for us. When we say, "I am good at characterization," we are automatically excluding something else.

This notion of identification can also seep into other aspects of our writing, such as our language choices. As a writer, it's important to remember that a word is a concept—it is fluid, not fixed. Even so, we often attach fixed definitions to concepts in our writing. We bring to the table all of our experiences of what "teacher" means. The scary fourth grade teacher with red hair in an impossible beehive and orange lipstick smudged across her front teeth. The bushy-mustached professor who embodied Chaucer so much you were able to at least tolerate the text. The teachers whose names you no longer remember. See how the word "teacher" is no longer an empty slate? Words and concepts have associations with readers. Each word (writer, teacher, fill in the blank) has its own baggage. This is the nature of our art form, so rather than work against it, work with it consciously. To do this, remember the cornerstone of specificity. Don't assume we see what you see. Don't assume we associate the same things (negative or positive) with a word or place that you do. Someone, somewhere, loves cauliflower. I do not. To assume I have cornered the worldview on cauliflower is to alienate my reader and do a disservice to my characters and to cauliflower.

By being aware that every word has its own associations (and that they aren't just your associations; each person has his or her own associations with words), you enter into a clarified space with language, your tool. From this place of clarity, not clutter, you can create your stories and characters.

Each day you come to your writing practice, approach it cleanly. No baggage. No expectations. No anticipations.

*Don't write today from your experience of writing yesterday.*
Take that in.

Don't write today from your experience of writing yesterday.

The moment you come to the blank page with the high of yesterday's writing, or the drudgery of yesterday's writing, you're clouding the present moment with needless clutter. Just because you hit one out of the park yesterday doesn't mean you will today. Just because you didn't, doesn't mean you won't. Release any attachments you have to those notions, and the time you spend writing—whether it's fifteen minutes or five hours—will be much more rewarding for you.

Don't get trapped by identification with a job, a style of writing, a way of storytelling. Be open. You don't know everything. You don't even know much—and that's the perfect place to write from. Once we think we "know" something, we often close the door on future information. Better to not know and be open than to know everything and be closed.

## CHAPTER 13

# Illusion of Control

This condition I call neither arising nor passing away, neither dying nor being born. It is without form and without change. It is the eternal, which never originates and never passes away. To find it is the end of sorrow.

—Udana Sutta

I t begins when you first try to write. You take your No. 2 soft lead pencil and make fresh marks on the newsprint theme paper. A looping *p* can turn into an *r*, which can become a *q*. If you never lift the lead from the paper, you can join them all together in a song of harmony and grace, but then you show the world what you have made and they tell you it is gibberish. The beautiful loops and lines you dragged from your heart are worthless.

So you learn, there is a way. There is a way to do things and a way not to do things. Your heart is sad, but you cover it up because when you make the loops and lines their way they smile at you and bring you juice. They tell you that you are smart and show your paper to other people. The juice is cold, sweet, and sticky.

It no longer matters that you cannot understand what you wrote because your letters are mirrors of theirs. You have allowed them to take control of your letters. It happens without your noticing. You learn subconsciously that others can control your writing, so, logically, you believe you can as well. Indeed, you should. You must. After all, it's how it's done, isn't it?

I worry a lot about rules. I want to stand in the right line, drive in the right lane, and say the right things. I was raised to believe that if you did the right things you'd be rewarded. I could see the benefit of not driving in the lane facing oncoming traffic. I could see it would be more efficient if only people with fewer than fifteen items went through the express checkout line. I do understand we have to communally agree on what a g is—what it looks like, what sounds it can make, what words it's a part of—in order to communicate. But I learned odd rules about writing in school, such as:

> Never begin a sentence with a conjunction.
>
> Never end a sentence with a preposition.
>
> Each new paragraph should begin with a transitional word.
>
> A paragraph contains five to seven sentences and always begins with a topic sentence.
>
> An essay's final paragraph must sum up all that has come before it.

These are odd things that have little to do with writing and much to do with constructing. Much to do with trying to control what's already written on the page. Much to do with teaching the student that writing is something that can be mastered, dominated, put in its proper box for its proper praise. Much to do with the killing of the writing spirit.

It's a hot day in Charlotte. I'm in the seventh grade. Our text is *Warriner's English Grammar*. My English teacher, Mrs. Peeler, is a formidable woman who also happens to attend our church. She is the clichéd English teacher—gray hair pulled back into a bun, glasses on a silver chain around her neck, red lipstick, which occasionally stained the surface of her teeth, and nude pantyhose and high heels, no matter how hot the day. She made us memorize poems and then come to the front of the class and recite them. I still remember mine. William Wordsworth's "Daffodils."

She taught us to diagram sentences (a miraculous feat that has somehow fallen out of favor), and with that, she showed me that every word in a sentence has a purpose. You could see in your diagram if you had too many modifiers for your noun or verb. You could see if the subject of the sentence had no object. You could revise it and make a brand-new structure, a brand-new picture. Most of the kids loathed diagramming, but I thought it provided a door into language I'd never walked through before. (Oops, there I go, ending a sentence with a preposition; oops, "before" is used as an adverb there. How does one keep it straight?) In order to diagram a sentence well, you had to communicate with the words themselves. You had to ask the adjective, "What are you modifying?" And the adjective would answer. You had to ask the prepositional phrase which verb it connected with. You had to listen to the words' answers. You couldn't just randomly assign words to each other. They simply wouldn't fit.

Contrary to what many students thought, I didn't think diagramming sentences force-fed rules down our throats. I thought diagramming sentences taught us to listen to the beauty of an individual sentence and, even deeper than that, taught us to focus on the importance of each word choice and ask ourselves, Does that word belong there? Is another word a better choice? If we take out the word, does the sentence change in meaning or aesthetics? We couldn't make those choices with our intellects. The choices came from our connections to the desires of the sentence itself.

How do we know what a sentence desires? We have to ask it. How does a sentence know what it desires? It asks the paragraph. And the paragraph? Well, yes, it asks the chapter. And the chapter must ask the work as a whole what it desires.

Huh? How the heck do you do that?

Remember when they told you how to write a paragraph? And they gave you rules such as don't start a sentence with "and." And they told you writing comes from somewhere *out there,* involving sources and citations and documentation. And they told you that there were nine patterns of development for your work, and that the thesis statement is the last sentence in the opening paragraph. They told you these things not because they're wrong or bad. They do, in fact, work, and they can help a student who has no interest in what language can do write a solid composition. But for a student who is a writer—for a student who loves what sentences do—the rules are the stones in the pockets of your jeans. They can both anchor and drown you. Clear out your mind so you stop hearing the rules before you hear the writing. When you don't know where to go next, look to the sentence you last wrote for clues. What does the verb denote? What image does the noun conjure up?

It's hard to know how much of these rules we've absorbed. It's also hard to know how much these rules control our writing, keeping us from exploring ideas and stories, or even from hearing our own voices. When I was seven, I went to visit my pediatrician, Dr. Huff, for my final dose of liquid polio vaccine. The doctor handed me the plastic packet of vaccine and told me to put it in my mouth. I did exactly that. A few minutes later he came back in the office. I still had the liquid in my mouth. He and my mother laughed at me.

"Why didn't you swallow it?" he asked.

I swallowed, but I was bewildered. "You didn't tell me to swallow it. You told me to put it in my mouth."

My literal interpretation of the doctor's instructions shows you how strongly I wanted to follow directions, how strongly I wanted to do everything right. How much I believed others had control. My ninth grade English teacher took off points if our cursive letters didn't have all the appropriate tails. If she couldn't tell our periods from our commas, she marked the whole sentence wrong. The church we belonged to taught me I was born in sin. My Southern culture taught me not to wear white after Labor Day and that a lady should always wear a hat.

"Why didn't you swallow it?" What a provocative question. I did swallow a lot of it. I swallowed rules and doctrines and fears and contradictions. But all that swallowing left little room for listening. When you take the time to be still and listen, the first things you'll hear are the things you swallowed into your belly. You'll hear the things you've absorbed over a lifetime. You'll hear the scratches of your mother's fears and your father's rage. You'll hear a chorus of uninvited voices in an avalanche of shoulds and shouldn'ts, dos and don'ts. Sit a while longer. What sounds and voices are yours underneath that din? The clanking of other people's agendas is enough to make many a writer get up and decide this gig isn't for him. Stay. What's under your mother's sadness? What's under your grandmother's alcoholism? What's under the programming of never beginning a sentence with "and"? The ideas you've swallowed built a wall. Shake it down. Move into your lungs and breathe; then break the sadness loose so it can float away.

Stay. Stay longer than you ever thought you could. Sit cross-legged or not. Sit in a chair or on the floor. Sit on your bed or in your car. But sit. Stay. Look at each thing you've swallowed and ask yourself: Is it mine? Does it serve me? Then ask yourself what you feel is the next step. Ask your body, not your mind. When we learn to shake off the rules that keep us from our true voice, when we sit long enough to hear where our story should go next, we're left with the challenge of writing. Here we're faced with another aspect of control—the ability to control an emotion or experience enough to express it on the page.

To attempt to write about an experience separates us from the actual experience. To attempt to use language, that two-dimensional abstract medium, to convey an emotion separates us from the emotion. To attempt to analyze an event, a thought, a feeling, pulls us farther and farther from our direct experience. To label a laugh, even with the five letters of the word "laugh," is to freeze it, mummify it, burden it with all our projections, expectations, and past experiences of laughing. The rigid spine of the letter *l*, the dip of the *au*, the tail of the *g*, boxed in by the chair of the *h* makes, when you dissect it, a bumpy outline of a sacred experience that bubbles up from the belly and escapes into the world from the cage of your bones.

Try to hold a laugh, a smile, a surprise sob. Try to hold the "I love you" that slips through your teeth, the "I miss you," the "thank you." Just try to wrap your fingers around such phrases. When you unclench your palm, you'll find nothing. Instead, rather than holding tightly to the rigidity of form, look softly for the laugh's essence. The pitter-patter of its feet across your tongue. The salt of its juice in your eyes. Any act of writing is an attempt to hold still what is by its nature moving, so that a reader can bring his or her own gentle spark to the words and put the scene in motion, complete with personal past experiences and conceptions about those words, thus making the magic that is a story.

How then, to write a laugh? If all we have are letters, then how can the expanse of a laugh be contained? If we are called to write, then what are we to do with a two-dimensional medium in a three-dimensional world?

To attempt to tell a reader what to think, feel, or do—to attempt to control a reader's response—will destroy the relationship between reader and author. Instead, step away from the podium. Sink into a comfortable chair, cross your legs, and open your ears, then listen inward and outward. Resist the urge to control the outcome, either of the writing or of reactions to it. Dictating the terms of receipt of your work creates a rigid structure that will cause readers to rebel.

Think about how you would feel in a prison cell. What would you be willing to listen to in a cage? Make a soft, cozy space instead. Give readers room. Accept that you cannot capture with 100 percent authenticity and accuracy the way your uncle laughed at knock-knock jokes. Move underneath the laugh and pay homage to its essence. Etch a specific detail into your paper. A specific sound. Try a comparison. If it's too much, pull back. Don't pile metaphor upon simile upon analogy. Ground us in the scene. Let the laugh dance through the action, its footsteps adding the soundtrack. Do this with a feather, not with a hammer. Do this with the precise verb, the exact color's hue. Do this without any expectation that readers will hear your uncle's exact laugh. Trust that the lightness and specificity of your language allowed the reader to be grounded—while she, with her inner ear, heard the laugh of her own uncle, and in that sacred place embraced you, open heart to open heart.

## CHAPTER 14

# Illusion of Distractions

It is crucial to know when it is appropriate to withdraw our attention from things that disturb our mind. However, if the only way we know how to deal with certain objects is to avoid them, there will be a severe limit as to how far our spiritual practice can take us.

—Lama Thubten Yeshe, *Introduction to Tantra*

My agent frequently tells me that no one is as good at finding distractions as writers. She's correct. In graduate school, one of my seminar instructors, Jo Ann Beard, talked about the dangers of the poppy field. You know the place, I'm sure. The pretty colored poppy field from *The Wizard of Oz* where Dorothy and her gang are almost to Oz—they can see the glittering Emerald City—and they decide they'll rest a while in the beautiful red poppy field. Before they know it, they've lost hours and hours of time.

My husband uses the term "cheese crumbs," from the book *Bonk*. The book compares the behavior of male and female rats during sexual intercourse. The male, apparently, is single-directionally focused. The female rat, not so much.

She's easily distracted by cheese crumbs. So my husband and I will be walking down the street, and I'll spot something shiny or flowy in a store window and stop midtracks to go inside. "Cheese crumbs," he'll say.

But aren't they yummy and wonderfully sparkly?

Shunryu Suzuki tells us that the most important thing we can do in this life is to remain in our chair with a quiet mind. Yet our mind is programmed to seek out the next thing—the biggest, brightest, shiniest thing. The newest diet fad. The newest truck. The newest home with the biggest pool. The desire gets us moving, but it gets us moving away from, rather than toward, what we thought we wanted. It gets us responding to endorphins, which feels great for the moment, and then, not so great. So we go searching for more cheese crumbs.

As writers, we must constantly ignore the cheese crumbs so we can actually get to the work of writing. Of course, we are good at turning our distractions into excuses. During any semester, I hear every excuse imaginable for not writing. I hear there's too much work in other classes. Too many hours at the day job. No inspiration. Too much inspiration. A computer crashed (um, pen and paper, anyone?). Too much time spent on the couch watching television or sitting at the computer.

Don't lose sight of the choices you make for managing your time. You don't have to check your Facebook page four times a day. You don't have to tweet or read a hundred industry blogs. You don't have to watch ten hours of *Battlestar Galactica* in a row. So pay attention. What are you doing? Don't berate yourself, just notice. How are you choosing to spend your time? Interestingly, it can also be easy to turn your writing into an addiction or a distraction.

Perhaps you can already see how these concepts are rooted in attachment and aversion. When you are attached to a distraction in your writing (which, of course, is an aversion to doing the writing), you stop the flow of the moment. You get stuck. If you're becoming obsessed over your writing practice and finding yourself slowly moving away from contact with friends and family, take notice. Pull back a little. Breathe. The middle path will give you more space to stretch. If you're too far left or too far right, you'll soon be backed into a corner. When you keep moving, you don't get stuck. If you're pulled and pushed by all the cheese crumbs (and this world is full of cheese crumbs!), you'll find the whole world overwhelming and exhausting.

Part of the illusion of the distraction lies not in the distraction itself, but in the promise of what the distraction will bring. The illusion also lies in the belief that distractions are inevitable. That there's no way not to succumb to twelve hours a day of television. There is. Notice the distractions most prevalent in your life. Stand up to them. Challenge them. You are the only one who can make yourself write. Television, overtime at work, no separate home office—these things are not keeping you from writing. They are simply elements of a life. Don't give them weight they don't deserve to carry.

A disciplined mind will put you on a disciplined path. Disciplined doesn't mean rigid and unyielding though. It simply means focused. A practice gives you a focus. A writing practice teaches you to release an attachment to an outcome. It teaches you to show up and be present, if only for five minutes. The more frequently you can embody presence and focus, the more likely you are to recognize when you fall out of it during your day (and we all do). The more focus you have, the less likely that cheese crumb distractions will call to you around every turn. It doesn't mean you'll never have a cup of coffee or stop for a glass of wine or buy a sparkly scarf. It does mean you won't be undone by those things and find yourself at the end of your days wondering what happened to all the time you thought you had.

## CHAPTER 15

# Illusion of Publication, Success, and Fame

A sage can have things without feeling he
"owns" them.
The sage does things without putting an
emotional stake into the outcome.
The task is accomplished,
but the sage doesn't seek credit or take pride
in the accomplishment.
Because the sage is not attached to the
accomplishment,
the accomplishment lasts forever.

—*Tao Te Ching*, chapter 2

Y ou'd have to be living in a cave not to be aware of the upheavals and challenges in the publishing industry. You can barely look at *Publisher's Weekly* these days without reading news of a publishing house closing, or consolidating, or laying off staff. Spend even a small amount of time in the blogosphere of editors, agents, and publishers' blogs and you'll find yourself wanting to run for the hills and take up anything but writing. You can read agent blogs that give you a rundown of their weekly stats—how many manuscripts received, how many rejected, how many requested. The odds are daunting, and yet, people keep giving it a shot.

I can't tell you what's going to happen with the book industry in ten years, or how many people are going to be reading books, or if we're all going to be reading e-books on our e-readers, or if somehow stories will be mind-melded to us, but I can tell you that you can waste a great deal of your energy worrying about what publishing might do. There are stories of authors garnering wide acclaim with their first books, but if sales don't reach the megamillion dollar mark, they may find themselves unable to sell a second book. There are stories of authors getting picked up, getting the advance, turning in the manuscript, only to find their editor has been laid off and no one else at the company is "passionate enough" about the story to take it on. You can read about release dates being pushed farther and farther out into the future, and publishers staking their entire season on big names like Dan Brown or J. K. Rowling.

Do not be discouraged, gentle ones. All this may be happening, but it doesn't have anything to do with you. If . . . (OK, are you ready for the big *If*?) . . . your sense of worth as a writer isn't hanging on what a publisher or agent might or might not do. What are you writing for? Whom are you writing for? Why are you writing in the first place?

Publishing is a business. Perhaps this is one of the hardest things for new writers to accept. The publishing world isn't waiting to nurture your career. It isn't waiting to take a chance on you. It's a business, and, for good or bad, it operates on a business model; namely, more money should come in than goes out. If you can make money for them, great. If your work doesn't make money, then thanks, but no thanks. I'm not going to tell you this doesn't suck, but I am going to tell you that you need to get over yourself and any sense of entitlement you might feel because you're the literary genius the world has been waiting for. No one's waiting. So what do you do? It's similar to the Buddhist question: what do you do when no one's watching? What do you write, how often do you write, how much do you push yourself with your craft if no one is waiting for your manuscript?

There's no right answer, as you might suspect, but it's worth exploring what your own answer might be. If your sense of self and your sense of worth as a writer hinge on getting a front-page review in the *New York Times* and an Oprah book pick, then you're setting yourself up for a lot of needless suffering. As writers, we naturally want to be read. We want our work to reach others. We want to communicate, reach an audience, and change the world, perhaps. I'm not knocking that at all. I feel it too. I want to reach millions of people. I want to be recognized. I want to be featured on blogs and followed on Facebook. I'm human. But I have to realize that fame isn't real. I have to ask myself what my authentic relationship with the work is, and it comes back all the time to my writing and me. That's the part that matters. I have to release my attachment to the rest.

Easy, right? I'll wave my magic writer's wand, and you'll no longer want an Oprah appearance, or the National Book Award, or a nod from the Pulitzer committee. You'll no longer want your novel to be the subject of an auction between Random House and Simon & Schuster. You'll no longer even want a big advance. Feel better now? Maybe you're at least smiling.

You cannot control the publishing industry. You cannot control which books get reviewed and which ones don't. You cannot control who reads your blog. You cannot control who will pick up your book at the bookstore and whether they will smile or put it down in disgust. When publication is your *only goal*, you are setting yourself up for a great deal of suffering. I'm not saying don't try to get your work published. I'm not saying you should stop doing due diligence to find out who might be the best audience for your work or stop working to make your writing as good as it can be. You can do all of those things. You can show up to do your writing practice. You can research appropriate markets. You can develop ways to self-promote your work. But you can't decide what Random House is going to pick up for the fall. Don't kid yourself; they don't know either. Trends are random. Trends often take the publisher by surprise. Don't write for what you think people will be buying in a few months. Remember that the publication schedule is usually about eighteen to twenty-four months from acquisition to book-in-hand unless you're the sole witness to the crime of the century or a general in a current war or a member of a recently ousted administration. If you're a new author or a midlist author, the tides of publishing are not rising and falling based on what you do. And, as hard as writing is, nothing is quite as hard as writing a book you don't care about—featuring a topic you came up with because you thought it would sell—and then, heaven forbid, you sell it and now have to write it and, frankly, could care less about. It'll show. The advance won't be enough money to undo the damage you're doing to your writing integrity.

Your responsibility is to your writing. Write what is within you to write and release the rest. Don't try to please the editor of the week. She might not be there next week. Write your novel or your memoir or your nonfiction book. Write your poems. Make them as good as you can make them. Send them out. When they get rejected, send them out again. Keep in this flow, and you'll be better able to remember that you are a writer, and that you are doing what you love and what is burning in your heart to do. There is great joy in that, and, believe it or not, there can be publication in that. There can be fame. But as quickly as those arrive, they vanish, and you'll find yourself chasing the illusive next greatest thing. It's a circle you'll never find your way out of until you stop chasing.

Let me say it again: the publishing industry is not waiting for you. Don't stop the flow of your own work by trying to please it. Don't make each rejection slip (and yes, Virginia, there will be rejection slips) a reason to stop or believe you're not good enough. There are as many reasons why a work is rejected as there are sands in the proverbial hourglass. Your responsibility is to your craft and to the voice of your work. Keep your eyes there. When publication happens, it will neither unmoor you nor freeze you. It will be just the next right thing.

## CHAPTER 16

# Illusion of Money

Materialistic knowledge can only provide a type of happiness that is dependent upon physical conditions. It cannot provide happiness that springs from inner development.

—His Holiness the Dalai Lama

Why include the subject of money in a book about writing? Listen to these comments:

"If I had enough money, I'd quit my job and write all day."

"If I had enough money to go to Europe for six months, I could finish my novel."

"If I had enough money to get my kids through school, then I could spend some time writing my book." (Notice that phrase, "spend some time." Another illusion. Another commodity.)

"I don't have enough money. I have to work three jobs just to make ends meet. I don't have any time to write."

Perhaps no other symbol in our culture holds as much promise and seduction as money. The stories of money associated with success within our cultural mythology as well as our individual mythology are powerful, and often unconscious. "Enough" money will make us happy. And it goes even deeper than that; it's not so much the money, but the things, the lifestyle, the partner, the car or home that the money can bring us. These things are, according to our cultural mythology, unattainable without money. The one-dollar bill—the piece of paper—isn't worth all that much as a piece of green paper. Where its value comes in is through our perception of what the piece of paper can bring us, the *story* associated with the symbol.

In college, my economics professor held up a one-dollar bill in class. "What would you be willing to do for this?" Turned out, not very much. Then he held up a twenty. "Now?" And finally, a hundred-dollar bill. It seemed like no one was willing, at least on the surface, to murder for a hundred dollars, but the exercise got the whole class thinking. "It's just a piece of paper," he said. "Just a piece of paper with a number on it. Would you kill for it? Would you steal for it? Would you risk your life for it?"

Stories about money hang in all of our closets. What does it mean to have money? What does it mean to be without money? Where does money fall on the "what is valuable in this family" rule book? What is money tainted with? Can it be clean? What perfect storm of events had to occur before money found its way into your account? Were you born into money? Do you feel guilty about having money? About not having money? How much of your psychic energy is spent worrying about money—how to get more of it, how to better manage what you have, how to save enough so you can retire one day or put your kids through college, how to have "enough," whatever enough means to you?

I'm not going to talk about the virtues of poverty, tell you to give all your money away, or suggest that once your mortgage payment is less than 15 percent of your take-home pay you'll be safe, happy, and at peace. I'm not about to tell you that life isn't a bit easier if you've got enough money for good food and a safe place to live. I will, however, encourage you to think about what your relationship with and beliefs around money *are,* and I want to show you an alternate way of thinking about money.

You might have worked your entire life and accumulated fifty thousand dollars for retirement. One day, you want to go to the bank to retrieve your money. They give you back your fifty thousand dollars, only you suddenly realize that that fifty grand isn't worth what you thought it was. The value of the dollar has shifted, and what you thought you had you no longer have, even if you actually have fifty thousand one-dollar bills in your hand. Think about currency exchange rates. One year you travel to Europe, and your money "goes farther" than it would in the United States. The next year, you need twice as many U.S. dollars to travel to Europe for the same vacation as you would have the month before. Go figure.

Let's go back to the example from my economics class and think about money as a symbol for a story. What story does one dollar get you? Now think about perspective and point of view. What story does one dollar get you if you're nine years old and it's 1943? What story does one dollar get you if your sole desire is a pack of peanut M&M's? See how story and symbol are connected to setting, place, and character motivation? What do you think one thousand dollars would give you? Ten thousand dollars? One hundred thousand dollars? Don't be ruled by your story of money, and don't put your writing life on hold waiting for big money. That's the illusion of money. Not that we don't need it. Not that it doesn't provide a service. Not that it isn't a tool. But it isn't the *answer.* It won't make you a writer.

When I went to graduate school, I was in a class with a fifty-something man. He was very excited about starting the program. He finally had enough money to take some time off from work and devote himself to writing. His kids were finished with college. His house payment was manageable. He was one of the most enthusiastic people about writing I'd ever met. But then he didn't come back one day. Or the next day. Or the next. Finally, we notified the program chair, who called his family, who also hadn't heard from him. We found out that he had died suddenly in his room, apparently of an asthma attack. He waited until everything was lined up for him to pursue what mattered to him. He had "enough" money. And then he died.

## CHAPTER 17

# You're Not the Only One

Every writer I know has trouble writing.

—Joseph Heller

When I was writing my first "real" novel in graduate school, my sea foam green iMac would power on by itself with its trademark "chung!" at 5:00 AM. I'd see the glow of the monitor under the closed office door from my bed. My coffee pot was programmed to start percolating at the same time. I had to be at my day job by 8:00 AM. It was a thirty-minute drive from my house to work. I needed an hour to shower, get ready, and eat breakfast. That meant if I actually got out of bed at 5:00 AM and went to my computer, I'd have ninety minutes to work before my day job began.

Theoretically, this was a perfect plan. I'd watched myself not writing. I'd watched myself talk about wanting to be writing, getting increasingly frustrated with each passing year that I wasn't writing nearly as much as I knew I should be. I saw my twenties passing before my eyes, and I believed that if I didn't make the best-seller list by the time I was thirty I'd have no chance at a writing career.

My best writing friend, Jeffrey, lived in San Francisco. He also had a day job. He also worried about his life passing too quickly. We both needed our day jobs. So we devised a phone-tree plan. We alternated weekday mornings calling each other at 5:30 AM. Just a quick call. "Are you writing? What are you working on today? Send me pages. Ciao." Some days we both were awake. Some days one of us woke up the other. Some days we forgot (or slept through). But most of the time we called each other. For a little over a year, we pulled each other out of bed, two thousand miles apart, and wrote. It was a trick, yes, but a trick that worked. It helped us both cultivate discipline. We didn't beat each other up when one of us forgot to call or when one of us was still in bed when the other called. We were each other's human muse, calling to gently poke the other awake.

Jeffrey died this past year, and of all the many things I miss about him, I miss his belief in my writing most of all. I miss his investment in me doing my work. I miss my investment in him doing his work. Sometimes I imagine those phone calls when I don't want to get out of bed. I imagine his voice. "Get up. What are you working on today? Send me pages. Ciao."

Given the chance, we writers will construct mountains in our paths toward finishing a book. What if you didn't get in your own way? What if you didn't wait for someone else to recognize your talent to start writing? What if you didn't wait for your current book to sell before starting that next novel?

You're not alone. We seem to need to build these mountains so we can learn the lessons of tearing them down. Watch yourself with a discerning eye. Be diligent. It takes a long time to build a mountain, but the pace of mountain building can be so slow that you don't notice what has happened until you realize you've got to somehow climb over that mountain. Remember, we aren't machines. It's not healthy for us to keep an absolute routine every day forever and ever amen.

Some days it's just not the right thing to work on your book. But only you can discern whether or not it's the right day, or if you're getting in your own way.

When we are in harmony, writing flows. When we compose a sentence, we follow one word after another until we reach the period. You know you've felt it, those moments (hours!) when time has no meaning. You're absorbed into the flow of language and your story. Moments like that are not the sole property of the unusually gifted. They aren't given only to the privileged few. They are yours when you get out of your own way.

Become a ruthless watcher of your own patterns. Learn what is habit and what is familiar. Recognizing your habits will help you recognize what is comfortable. The trap of comfort hides many a self-sabotaging agent.

Be wary of all-or-nothing thought patterns. An example: if I don't write at least two thousand words today, I'm never going to finish this book. If you write two hundred words a day for ten days, you'll get your two thousand words. If you write two hundred words a week, in ten weeks you'll get your two thousand words. The slow and steady pace gets you to the next level.

Don't slip into the easy cloak of needing validation from an outside source. I didn't *need* Jeffrey to call me at 5:30 in the morning. I believed I did, but I didn't. I thought I needed someone else to be invested in my work for it to matter. It's great when someone else is invested in your work, but it isn't required.

Don't identify with the trap of writer's block. Writer's block is not a concrete thing. It is a concept, which means it's fluid, and you can accept it or not. Don't accept it. Your writing is never blocked. You just have not found the way to access your writing, but you will. Just like you are your own best teacher, you are your own worst enemy.

Be realistic about your lifestyle. If you're not willing to give up four hours of television at night, then be OK with that. Don't curse the writing gods for not providing you writing time. You had the time. You made other choices. No harm, no foul. If you're currently juggling three jobs and four children, be realistic about the odds of you getting a solid week off from everything to write (and if you had that, wouldn't you probably crash on the couch for half of it?). Instead, find small blocks of time (a block of time can be five focused minutes) in which you maintain your relationship with your writing. Fighting with your life's responsibilities is a bit like fighting with your body. Some of us get to be size three. Some of us don't. Why fight what can't be changed? If you're raising children, you're raising children. Work *with that* rather than against it. If a trust fund with a handsome butler named Sergio is not a part of your life, join the club and stop wishing for that scenario to occur before you start writing. Sergio, sadly, isn't on his way. Work with your assets and liabilities. Wishing they were something other than what they are will cause you suffering. And besides, that handsome butler named Sergio is no doubt a capital *D* distraction anyway!

Don't worry about the end result. Don't agonize over how to write a query letter until you've written and revised your book. It's important to write a good query letter, but it's pointless until you've written a manuscript. Don't put publication concerns before craft concerns. Learn your craft. Write the best book possible. Then do the next right thing.

Be cognizant of stagnation, which doesn't always manifest itself in sloth. Think of stagnation as any behavior, routine, or pattern that has solidified. This can be anything, from what appears on the surface to be lazy (spending fifteen hours a day in bed on the weekend) to what appears to be very industrious (a disciplined writing schedule of 6:00

to 8:00 AM, Monday through Friday). Rigidity and stagnation block the flow of energy in your body, which will in turn block the flow of energy in your writing. The shaking practice I introduced you to will help you release these areas of stagnation and rigidity in your body.

Know thyself. Remember, only you know in your heart of hearts if it's the right time to watch that episode of *Battlestar Galactica* or if it's the right time to finish that chapter. It'll take some practice (I still work on this) to recognize what the truth of the moment is. Be gentle as your awareness deepens.

You'll find, as your relationship with your writing becomes softer and more consistent, that the voice on the other end of the 5:30 AM telephone call is your writing. *Hey. How's it going today? Send me some pages. Ciao.*

# THE WRITING WARRIOR PRACTICE

Failure happens all the time. It happens every day
in practice. What makes you better is how you react
to it.

—Mia Hamm

art 3, Dissolving Your Illusions, introduced you to
the Writer's Wheel of Suffering. Perhaps many of the
illusions on the wheel were familiar to you. Perhaps
not. Please don't agonize over whether or not you're suffering enough to be a writer! That's not the objective here. The
intention of this section is to help you see common obstacles
in a writer's life. As a Writing Warrior, first you must see
with clarity and compassion what is in your way. Only then
can you make the best choices about what to do next. Awareness is a profound gift.

As your awareness deepens, so might your resistance.
This is common. Return to the practice: the breath, the shaking, the writing. Show up especially when you don't want to.
The work you're doing may not be apparent to you right now,
but it is occurring, breath by breath, word by word.

## INTERNAL CONVERSATIONS

*You can use these internal conversation exercises for personal work. The deeper your relationship with yourself, the deeper your writing becomes. Feel free to use poetry or prose to respond.*

The Illusion of Time: What is your relationship with time? Fill in the blank with a verb: "I am always _____ time." Trust your intuition on this one. Go further and ask for clarification on that verb. For example, if you wrote *I am always chasing time,* ask yourself to be more specific about the word *chasing.* Don't judge your word choices. Just notice. What can shift in your life to alter your current relationship with time?

The Illusion of Thoughts: Spend ten minutes just writing your thoughts as they surface and pass through your mind. Can you catch one with no effort? As each thought appears, another one is forming like waves in the ocean. Don't try to hold back the ocean. Merge with it instead.

The Illusion of What a Writer Is: Ask yourself what you think a writer is. Free write as long as you need to until you reach a natural end point. Are these helpful beliefs or are they getting in your way? What beliefs can be rewritten? Can you see yourself as a writer? William Faulkner said, "Don't be a writer. Be writing." Spend some time journaling around that quotation. Remember, a writer is someone who writes. Nothing more. Nothing less.

The Illusion of Identification: What areas of your writing do you overidentify with? You might try drawing a table and filling in the legs of that table with those areas. What is missing? Is your table lopsided? What areas of your writing are you afraid of or avoiding?

The Illusion of Control: Free write beginning with this phrase: *Losing control means . . .* Then, *Being in control means . . .* How much energy do you spend trying to be in control and trying to avoid being out of control? What do you associate with being out of control? With being in control?

The Illusion of Distractions: Make a list of everything that distracts you during the day from your tasks. (The tasks don't have to be writing.) Practice self-observation without judgment. Simply being aware of what distracts you will begin a subtle shift in your ability to remain present.

The Illusion of Publication, Success, and Fame: The more educated you are about the publishing process and the more knowledge and practice you have working with your craft, the better your chance of attaining publication. Research the blogs of agents, editors, and other writers. Be realistic and sensible. Don't use this process as a substitute for actually writing. Writing comes first. Without that, there's nothing to publish.

The Illusion of Money: Money, like time, is something we have to learn to work with. What belief systems do you have around money? You might begin with this phrase: *If I had enough money, I'd . . .* Or, *People who have money are . . .* Or, *My relationship to money is . . .*

---

WRITE NOW

*The following exercises can be applied to works in progress or used as prewriting. Feel free to use poetry or prose to respond.*

Write a scene in which your character betrays something or someone that is an integral part of his or her life. What are the consequences?

Take a character you're having trouble with. Examine the character's relationship with control. Put that character in a situation where he or she is out of his or her element. What happens?

Examine your characters' relationships with money. You might start with describing the contents of a wallet or purse. What myths or stories does your character have around money? For example, does your character always have a twenty-dollar bill in his or her wallet out of fear that the ATM will be out of cash? Where does money fall on your character's value scale?

Make a list of all the things getting in the way of your character achieving his or her goals. What distraction does your character face along the way? What are the gifts of that distraction? What are the costs? How long has the distraction been a part of your character's life? How did it begin? What need is it filling? What would it take to let it go?

Choose a character who seems to be stuck in a current piece of your writing. Whose voice does this character wish to hear on the other end of the phone? Why? Write a dialogue between the character and the voice.

PART FOUR

# Committing to Your Authentic Path

## CHAPTER 18

# Self-Observation
# without Judgment

Let's trade in all our judging for appreciating. Let's
lay down our righteousness and just be together.

—Ram Dass

L et's start with a koan.

One day Banzan was walking through a market.
He overheard a customer say to the butcher, "Give
me the best piece of meat you have."

"Everything in my shop is the best," replied the butcher.
"You can not find any piece of meat that is not the best." At
these words, Banzan was enlightened.

We make judgments every day. We compare ourselves to
others and our writing to other people's novels, poems, and
stories. We make negative statements: "My story is boring."
"I can't write." "That novel is better than mine." These judgments on their own are not helpful. We need to look deeper
into these statements. Why do you feel this way? What does
this reveal about yourself? How can you respond to make
your work better? When we open ourselves up to observing

the root of our judgments, we'll soon see that everything in our shop is the best because everything is 100 percent what it is. Honoring the perfection of each step in your writing process helps you to see that all of your flaws help you deepen your craft.

Each step, from prewriting, to outlining, to drafting, to starting over, to editing is perfectly itself. Why should your first draft be held to the standards of a final draft? Why can't that first draft simply be a perfect first draft? Why is it so difficult to look at our writing without picking apart everything that is wrong (or that we perceive to be wrong)? The world seems to tell us to compare ourselves to everyone and everything.

Let's return to the koan and examine the nature of "best" when it's not used in a comparative way. Each item in the butcher's shop is best because it is perfectly what it is. The piece missing from many people's thinking is the awareness that nothing is the same as anything else. No two pieces of meat are the same. No two people's writing journeys are the same. No two people's abilities are the same, and no two versions of a story are the same. Don't compare one to the other. Instead, examine the gifts that each one presents. Seeing what isn't working is not a flaw. It's a gift. Your first draft will not be like your second draft, yet each draft is complete unto itself. One is not trash while the other is brilliant. When you can call a first draft a first draft and be OK with that, you create space around yourself and your writing. When you view a first draft as something that failed to be a final draft, which is not in its nature to be, you create contraction.

Here's the trick. Look at yourself honestly without turning your judgment inward. Stop at the observation. Don't turn that observation, which is a powerful and important step toward self-awareness, into a judgment spiral. Don't use it to reconfirm a belief that you're worthless, selfish, a bad writer, or afraid. Don't use it to beat yourself up. If you view the things you find out about yourself and your writing as tools toward greater understanding, rather than ways to reinforce your negative self-talk, then you'll find you're a few steps ahead of the game in understanding self-observation without judgment. If you can avoid attaching an identifier to your behavior (for example, I am selfish), and if you can look without judgment at your behavior, then you're standing in a place of balance and harmony with what is.

For all the concepts we're discussing in this book, learning to work with them in one aspect of your life will make them available to you in other parts of your life. Once you begin actively cultivating self-observation without judgment in your writing life, you'll find it's impossible to turn it off in other parts of your life.

In writing classes, I see two primary ways that students judge themselves:

1. They compare their own work to the work of everyone else in the class, or for that matter, everyone else who ever wrote a book.
2. They compare their current writing to where they *think* they should be in their development.

Both of these ideas get in the way of authentic growth in your writing. The first example is easier to recognize and work with. The second example requires a significantly deeper willingness to work with the self.

Let's look at the first self-judgment. If you've never been in a situation where your work has been shared publicly, a writing class or a workshop presents a lot of opportunities to do so. Maybe you were the phenom of your high school English class and your teachers showered you with praise. Maybe you have dyslexia and were always told you would never be able to be a writer. Either way, you compared yourself to other writers. Leave your baggage about writing (and how others write) at the door. Come to a writing class or a writing project as empty as possible. Otherwise, your stories about yourself will weigh you down so much, the stories within you won't be able to fly.

The first time a class or critique group reads each other's work is a fabulous opportunity for practicing self-awareness. Were you so awed by everyone's talent that you felt unworthy to be in the group? Were you so appalled by the stories that you felt too advanced to be in the group? Did you begin right away by comparing your work with other people's work?

It's natural to do this, and one of the best ways we learn to make our craft better is by studying powerfully written work. Your class will likely have a participant or two who is farther along in their practice than you are. There will likely be a participant or two who is just beginning. There will definitely be people writing in all genres, which will present another opportunity for you to exercise self-observation without judgment. Do you "hate" fantasy writing? Mysteries? Thrillers? Literary fiction? Not any more. Drop those labels and read what your classmates are writing. We've all got literary preferences, but those preferences don't matter when it comes to learning about writing. They're an artificial barrier between you and the work.

Maybe you're one of those students who's too shy to present your work to the class because another student is so brilliant and you're so, well, not so brilliant. Take a deep breath and get over your sweet self. Stand behind your work at whatever stage it's in. If you're a parent, are you embarrassed to have your three-year-old child interact with a twelve-year-old child because they're at different developmental stages? Writing is the same. It has an infancy, a terrible twos phase, a gawky adolescence (sometimes many years of gawky adolescence), a young adulthood filled with mistakes, and finally a maturity that is still not perfect (check out those lines under your eyes) but is complete. You won't write a perfect book. You won't even write an almost-perfect book. You can write the best book you're capable of at the time you write it. I would hope that what I wrote in my twenties is significantly different from what I wrote in my thirties. Now that I'm in my forties, I want to keep pushing myself, keep trying new things, keep stretching the limits of what I know (or think I know) about writing. If I don't maintain this flow, I'll get bogged down and before too long I'll turn into the stodgy old professor who is stuck in some previous glory-filled decade, refusing to embrace the natural morphing of language and storytelling over time. I don't want to be that person, so I must be diligent about continual learning.

You've no doubt heard the concept of *beginner's mind*. A beginner's mind observes everything. It doesn't shut out what it thinks it already knows. It doesn't shut out what it thinks it will never need. It doesn't discount something because it doesn't like the person who said it. The beginner's mind is nonjudgmental, empty, and therefore available for anything. The longer you write and study writing, the harder it can be to maintain your beginner's mind. There's now junk in the way; perhaps you've completed a twenty-five thousand-dollar graduate program, or published four books, or won an esteemed prize. The junk from all these experiences is *only valuable in the degree to which you don't attach to it.*

Knowing things is great. Understanding the primary types of dialogue is great. Recognizing the key components of plot is great. But be wary of relying on your knowledge exclusively. If you do this, you might dismiss out of hand something that could really push your writing to the next level. If you're too attached to having an MFA, or a book deal, then you're viewing everything that comes your way through that filter. Practice saying, without judgment, "I don't know."

Say it over and over. I don't know. I don't know. I don't know. When you come to a workshop, when you critique a fellow student's manuscript, when you listen to comments on your own work, the mantra stays the same: *I don't know.* This will create space. When you have space, you have movement. When you have movement, you have growth. You don't have to act on the suggestion that you turn your historical romance into a crime novel starring three-eyed green octopus people, but listening to that idea might trigger something useful.

The second way students judge themselves, against their expectations of where they should be, is a bit more tangled. Listen honestly to this. Does anything sound familiar? You're forty-five years old. You should be able to catch on to this writing thing immediately. You should be able to download the information and then regurgitate beautiful sentences and compelling stories after three weeks of instruction, without having had to develop a previous writing practice. If you can't do this right away, then you're obviously not cut out to be a writer. This may sound harsh, but self-judgment is harsh. It's mean, nasty, and unrelenting. I want you to recognize it, so you can laugh at it rather than listen to it. I see it paralyzing too many students.

If you wanted to dance with the New York City Ballet, do you think you could audition tomorrow, be selected, and then be performing next week if you had never taken a ballet class, never performed before, and, no, never squished your toes into those pointe shoes? Yet people show up to writing classes every year thinking they can "learn it all" and then go forth and produce. Dancers practice. Athletes practice. Writers practice. The folk wisdom is that it takes about ten to fifteen years of practice to find your voice and rhythm as a writer. That's fifteen years of actually writing. That's a lot of writing. Journals. Stories. Practice novels. Essays. It's also sending work out and getting mostly rejections, but a few acceptances along the way, which shine light into your heart. Please hear what I'm saying so you are not ungrounded when these judgment thoughts pass through. Let them pass.

Writing is both an art and a craft, and even a lifetime's effort does not guarantee mastery. But you have more than enough time to form an intimate relationship with writing. You just have to decide how much work you will put into it. Only you. Don't sit on a mountaintop waiting for the muse to strike. The muse shows up when you show up, not the other way around.

Writing a good solid scene is a miraculous thing. Getting one sentence to sing, or one character to move another's heart, well, yeah, that's a lot. If you are in the direct experience—I am writing my novel. I am writing Cassandra's scene. She's about to slip on the banana peel—stay there. Stay in the story. Stay in the character. Don't jump forward into what you think you ought to be writing (it's only a speculation anyway, not where you are now).

If you find you're falling into this second camp of self-judgment, contrasting your work with what you believe it should be at this stage, then try thinking about why you have such unrealistic expectations for yourself. Pay attention to me here; I'm not telling you not to write well. I'm not telling you that you can't write well, or shouldn't write well. I'm just telling you to place some perspective on the whole puzzle. Release your desire for results, and for some reason (truly unbeknownst to me), you'll find yourself writing a lot. Writing better. Pushing yourself. It's the flow within the present moment that gives your writing what it needs to sustain itself. When you leave your body and let your mind go wandering in the shoulda/coulda/woulda/if only land, your writing will freeze up. It might even run away for a while.

This writing thing is challenging enough without you getting in your own way.

Be OK with where you are, with how your work is developing, while at the same time continuing to ask yourself the hard questions. Don't be OK with good enough. Don't be OK with an easy word choice, a simple plot construction. See what happens when you push yourself, when you trust yourself to try something new. When you release your attachment to the result, you'll be freer within yourself to experiment. It's these experiments that show you your authentic voice, not the canned responses you've been trained to give in school or at work. When you follow the path of your own intuition—what if I wrote this whole chapter in sentences that start with *A*—you'll find your own voice. You may decide it just doesn't work to start every sentence with *A,* but you'll have learned something. Perhaps most important, you'll have discovered that it's OK to try something new. It's OK for that attempt not to work. And it's OK to try something different, or even the same thing again later on (because we all know it never turns out exactly the same). Let there be a lightness and a sense of play in your writing practice. You'll notice an easing in your shoulders, a deepening of your breath, and a significant shift in your relationship with your work.

The way to transform judgment into a powerful tool is through observation. We need to continually observe our own writing. The key to effective observation is specificity. For example: my story needs a driving question. That's a statement. It provides information that will help my writing. Notice how different that is from saying: my story is boring. Specificity not only will help you see your work more clearly, it will remove the commentary that can be so devastating to a writer.

Think about adverbs. She cried. That's a statement. She

cried loudly. The adverb attaches a judgment to the sound, and that judgment requires qualification. Louder than what? Louder than all the noise in Grand Central station? Louder than the wind blowing through an empty lot? Louder than the person next to her? Judgments do the same thing as adverbs. They attempt to control a reaction and a response. When you control yourself this way, you stay stuck.

Lately we've become accustomed to judging many things in our lives. We can rate blog posts. Books. Music. Items of clothing we buy. YouTube videos. There's an opportunity for us to judge with a five-star system just about everything we consume. Do someone's comments help you better listen to a piece of music? Do they help you see something in a new light? Every once in a while, a comment does make a difference, and it's the comment that's specific. The comment that states exactly what worked and what didn't and why. This provides concrete information we can use to make our own choices. We're not responding to "that sucked" or "that's the most amazing thing ever." We're responding to specificity. Specificity allows us to grow and expand our own sphere.

Practice a discerning eye to determine the difference between a fact and a judgment. A statement such as *My protagonist is missing a desire* is a fact. There's nothing good or bad about it. It's an observation. However, a statement such as *My story says nothing of value* is a judgment. Judgments direct our thinking, taking away the power of direct experience. If you tell yourself your story says nothing of value, that is the lens through which you view your story as you try to revise it. That lens will prevent you from seeing what the story does say (and everything says something). Please don't freeze up before you even start moving. When you catch yourself judging yourself or others, just notice. Find the specificity underneath the judgment. Does it hold water?

How can you rephrase it? Don't beat yourself up. We're all human.

Under this big umbrella of self-observation without judgment, let's look at the role of a teacher or mentor in your development. We have all had them. In order to continue practicing beginner's mind, it's healthy to keep finding mentors and teachers in a wide variety of places, not just in your writing life. New people provide new perspectives. Take care, though, to avoid attaching too much importance to one teacher or one set of guidelines. For example, I see many students extremely attached to whatever the latest writer's magazine article says about character construction. They follow the steps with zeal. They cannot be swayed, it seems, to consider other ways of creating a character. Remember, no one person has the universal answer to anything. No scholar in any field is the definitive authority.

Be careful of transferring your dreams onto the shoulders of a teacher (and I say this both as a student and a teacher). When you attend a class, don't expect to simply open your brain and get the information you need downloaded. Don't be passive. Be an active participant in your learning and be open to all that's around you. Trust yourself to take what's of value and let the rest go.

Most teachers are genuine, compassionate, and interested in helping their students. This doesn't mean they're infallible, and it doesn't mean they're the right fit for you at all levels of your career. When something in a class isn't valuable to you, it may be the exact thing the student next to you needed to hear. That's one of the most confounding things about teaching; you'll never succeed every time with every student because no two students are the same. The best we can do is put forth authentic effort.

Don't look for the teacher who will fix everything for you, the teacher who will open the doors to publishing or to your heart. That projection is unhealthy for both you and the instructor. It will result in expectations that cannot be met, which will result in suffering, which will result in you not garnering any value from the instructor. No one else is responsible for you. No one else is going to write your book. No one is going to stand over you, saying, "Read, read, read! Write, write, write!" You've got to be your own first, best teacher. Engage the assistance of others, those whose styles you gel with and those who make you squirm. There is always an opportunity to learn, provided you don't close the door to your own growth. Remember: the teacher only makes the space. You must chart your own course.

## CHAPTER 19

# Absolute Vulnerability

Find out what you're afraid of and go live there.

—Chuck Palahniuk

I f you ever need to quickly clear a room of people, write the words "absolute vulnerability" on the board, smile at them, and say, "This is our objective for the entire semester." I did this recently in a memoir class I was teaching, and I truthfully didn't realize the powerful effects of that simple phrase on a group of writers. Some had a deer-in-the-headlights look. Others were chomping at the bit to "go there." Still others were calculating whether or not they could still get their money back for the course. True to their warrior nature, they stuck it out for sixteen weeks and emerged, changed, on the other side.

People often think writing is only about grammar and craft components and publishing. It's about how to make sentences clear and how to arrange events in a plot to make a story compelling. It's about a dramatic arc and an explosion of a scene from dry summary to powerful dramatization. But it most definitely is not about absolute vulnerability (whatever that means).

Discussions of craft components, while important, are

the intellectual aspect of the writing process, not the body-based one. Taking commas in or out is simply rearranging ships on the ocean of the story. What my writing students want to know, and what I want to know as well, is how to create the ocean. A monkey can eventually arrange the ships in an order that will produce a desired result. But creating the ocean, well, that's another matter entirely.

So the writer's job is to first find the ocean. And once you do find it, you must release the intellectual exercises and see what happens when you leap, naked, into the cold water. The more you know about what's going on in the ocean, the better your can position your writing and your life. The trouble is, most of us would rather stay as far away as possible from the churning waters. We'd rather etch our letters on the safety and predictability of dry land, thank you very much.

To write well, you have to bear unflinching witness to yourself as a character in your own story, regardless of whether you are writing fiction or memoir or poetry. You have to recognize that you are bringing up things from your murky depths *even if you don't know what they are.* You don't have to know everything. You have to trust the work and trust that you can bear witness to whatever emerges. To attempt to make art out of the slippery material of a life means you dive off the boat into the waters and trust that your absolute vulnerability brings out the vulnerability of everyone you're going to meet down there. Your vulnerability, your willingness to be naked, connects others with your work.

This is what authentic writing does: It pulls you from your comfortable fuzzy chair (or podium) of understanding the elements of narrative and how stories work, and it brings you face to face with the one thing you've buried under your avalanche of degrees and fictions. It traps you in, holds your eyelids open à la *Clockwork Orange* and says, "OK, baby. Tell me what you see." At first, you hem and haw and theorize and analyze and attempt to concretize, but after a while, your eyeballs ache from staring and you just surrender because at that point you have no other choice. That thing is there. In front of you. You can't pretend you don't see it. You can't pretend it doesn't see you. There's nothing left in the world now but you and that thing that you've been consciously not seeing all of your life.

"I am the story," it says. And you don't believe it because you can't see the narrative arc, and you wonder about the drama, and you realize you have not had the most dramatic of lives, and so you try to swim back to the surface, but your eyelids are still pried apart and you are strapped to the chair anyway, and really, now, you're a little curious. That's a quality all writers have. Without it, we spout the same stuff from book to book. With it, we reinvent, revise, and restructure all the time.

"All right," you say. "Tell me the story." And you listen, and you take notes, and you are grateful, in spite of your burning eyeballs and exhausted writing arm; you are grateful because nothing less than magic has occurred.

Recently, I had to surrender and listen to the story that was emerging. The image that occurred for me was a yellow swing. When it came to me the first time, I saw no inherent story there. Just a sweet memory of a little girl who used to think she could fly. But it kept coming back. The cheap plastic of the swing. Its Big Bird yellow color. The sheets on the clothesline nearby. The neighbor's bulldog, Tony. The clouds with their incessant swirling, their movement enough joy for anyone in a lifetime. I began to notice more: the neon yellow and green colors in the ropes that held the swing, wrapped four times and nailed to a scrap piece of lumber; the tiny holes in the seat, delightful because I could feel the air from my flight on the backs of my legs; my mother singing *Zip-a-dee-doo-dah* while she put the wooden clothespins on the sheets.

And then I saw, or didn't see, the story. The swing was empty. It was moving, sure, higher and higher, but no one was on it. No mousy-haired girl with too-green eyes. No laughing girl who found even the slickness of her tongue on her own teeth astonishing. No singing girl, who hadn't yet been told she couldn't sing. And that was it. Where did she go? Why did she go? Can she come back? These were the narrative questions.

And the answer was a story.

We've talked about direct experience and cultivating discipline to stay in the chair when faced with our inner selves. The next step involves giving ourselves permission to be vulnerable on the page. Think for a minute about the phrase "absolute vulnerability." What comes up for you? Often, one of the things that comes up for people is a primal fear for survival. After all, we can't survive in the big, bad scary world out there if we are absolutely vulnerable, right? We can't protect ourselves, our property, our families. Can we? Can we protect ourselves if we dare to splay ourselves open on the page? What happens if we dredge up everything on paper? Who will be left to keep us safe? We'll go into more in-depth work at the end of this section, but I think in order for you to get the most out of what you're reading now, it would be helpful to spend a few minutes journaling about absolute vulnerability. Go ahead and write. I'll wait.

OK. What did you find out?

Let's keep going. Think of an image or two of absolute vulnerability. Go beyond the cliché of a newborn infant or other cute baby animal. Don't be lazy here. The images and ideas you come up with can help stabilize you throughout your writing journey. The images will provide something concrete for you to hold on to as you move deeper into absolute vulnerability. They can anchor you. After you have a few images in mind, question yourself even further. What about these images evokes absolute vulnerability for you? And, upon further contemplation, would you say your assessments are accurate or just familiar? Let's pause here—accurate or familiar? Our conditioning leads to the way we experience situations and emotions. How many times will you refuse to eat a certain food or wear a certain type of clothing because you "know" what it will be like? How many relationships have you turned away from? How many job opportunities? How many story ideas? Begin to notice how the way you assume things will unfold affects the choices that you make. How often do you do that when you're writing? Do you assume too much knowledge about a story's arc? So much so that you can't allow your characters to move according to their own rhythms? (Notice I said *their own rhythms,* not yours.) Finally, how do these images of absolute vulnerability relate to your own feelings of absolute vulnerability?

Let's break down absolute vulnerability into some manageable chunks. What's the first thing you notice about that phrase? For me, it's the word "absolute." Suddenly, with that single qualifier, there's no room to hide; that word by itself is often pretty frightening for people. The word "absolute" is also interesting because it puts you face to face with yourself and your own capacity for truth-telling *and* for telling yourself a line of crap that poses as truth. There's no Absolute Vulnerability Police Force out there watching you. "No, she's not there yet. Just a little more! A little more!" There's also no end to how deep that word can go. What might be absolute today may travel a little deeper in six months. Both are authentic.

Absolute vulnerability means opening yourself up. Perhaps a better way of phrasing it is *letting things go.* You let your masks go. Your suits of armor. Your persona of who you think you ought to be, or who you think others believe you to be. You trust the impermanence of each moment enough to realize that any barrier between you and your direct experience will only mute your quality of life. You trust that you are stable and grounded enough that your center will not be swayed by whatever events pass through your sphere. You are able to be open because you know that you are not your body, not your thoughts, not your relationships. You trust in your ability to make decisions and to respond to situations with clarity and compassion.

Novelist Erica Jong says, "No one ever found wisdom without also being a fool. Writers, alas, have to be fools in public, while the rest of the human race can cover its tracks." Writers have to put it all out and let it flap in the breeze, not knowing whether anyone will see their work, like it, hate it, try to destroy it, or give it a prize. A Writing Warrior stands solidly in absolute vulnerability, unattached to any outcome. You give the reader your heart, with no conditions. Writing with no conditions is a gift. Writing with conditions is an obligation, and an ultimate source of suffering. Don't write to heal the world. Don't write to get back at someone, or to make up with someone. Use your personal journal for any type of writing you need to do to unburden your heart, but when it comes to creating art, write an honest, authentic story with no agenda except the terms the story dictates. Notice how clean it feels to be in this level of balance with your work.

Absolute vulnerability involves an intimacy with the self. The what? Yeah, I know. It just gets freakier. How do we cultivate an intimacy with the self? We return to direct experience. Zen master Dogen tells us, "Enlightenment is just intimacy with all things." Love that word "just" in there! He makes it sound so simple. As you move deeper into a place of self-observation without judgment, you will find this intimacy bubbling to the surface. You will notice your gaze naturally softening, both inwardly and outwardly, as the blanket of compassion wraps itself around you.

CHAPTER 20

# Soft Eyes

Be soft, even if you stand to get squashed.

—E. M. Forster

P lease take a minute to move into a space you find appealing. It can be inside or outside. Take your journal and a pen with you. When you arrive, find a comfortable seat, either on a chair or on the floor. If you're in a chair, rest both your feet flat on the floor. Breathe deeply into your belly three times. Exhale fully each time.

Now soften your body, your shell. Soften your gaze and then close your eyes. Soften your shoulders, your spine, your hips. Soften your breath so it sinks to your belly. Relax your tongue, your jaw, your throat. Relax your ears, your skull, your wrists, your fingers. Soften your mind. Allow your thoughts to pass through without clamping onto them. Release your eye sockets, your eyelids. Relax your teeth, your bones, your belly.

Your sweet, sweet belly.

Place your hands on your belly and feel it expand as you inhale, then feel it release on your exhale. Settle a little deeper into your hip bones. Keep breathing, your breath sinking, sinking into your belly. Your belly is fleshy and soft under your palms. Keep your hands on your belly. A lot of emotion is stored in the belly. You may want to run away from your belly energy. Stay. Stay with it, your awareness moving deeper inward, into your body and into your heart.

What do you notice? Is this a familiar place? Foreign? Frightening? Do you notice yourself fidgeting? Sit for a while, just observing, hands on your belly, breath moving deeper and deeper, slower and slower, fuller and fuller. Allow your exhale to be as long as your inhale. Soften, soften, soften.

Stay here as long as you like before continuing with this chapter. When you decide to move forward, notice the nature of your thoughts and breathing as you proceed. Just notice; don't judge.

Now slowly open your eyes and allow your gaze to travel around your space. Don't linger too long on any one thing or area. Imagine your gaze is softly stroking your environment. Rather than using your eyes as arrows to pinpoint a particular object or person, allow the edges of your vision to become slightly fuzzy. I find this is easiest to do when I consciously relax my jaw and tongue. You might want to allow the tip of your tongue to rest on the back of your tooth ridge. This is a grounding place. Keep your breath moving fully throughout your body.

When you're ready, take out your journal and begin writing down your thoughts. Practice just being in the flow with them. Don't try to make them *say* anything of deep importance. You might want to record other impressions, not just of what you see but of what you might smell. Do you notice any changes within your own mouth? A shift in the quality of the saliva? (I'm not making this up!) Are you more aware of any particular sensation in your body? No judgment. Just observation.

When you feel complete here, move on intuitively to something else. It doesn't matter what you pay attention to next, so long as it's something specific. Perhaps you want to follow a feeling that arose to see where it lands or where its source may be. Perhaps you want to move deeper into a sensation within your body, or explore an object in your field of vision more fully. Follow your thoughts. Once again allow them to pass through without judgment or attachment. This time, if you (when you) find yourself traveling away from the initial prompt, redirect yourself back to your original intention. Begin again. If you (when you) find yourself traveling away once again, redirect. Begin again. Redirect yourself at least three times before you allow yourself to move onto another subject. Continue in this pattern as long as feels right for you today. When you feel complete, record your thoughts. Then set your journal down, return your hands to your belly, and close with three deep breaths, inhaling and exhaling equally.

OK. What did we just do? Quite a lot actually. First, we placed ourselves in an environment in which we feel comfortable. Then, we concentrated our attention inward. We grounded ourselves by keeping our feet flat on the floor and by consciously directing our breath deep into the belly. Our hands on our bellies kept us connected to our source. By concentrating on softening, releasing, relaxing, letting go—whatever phrase you like—we are creating space. Where there's rigidity, there's tension. Where there's softness, there's release.

For many of us, the act of writing involves a lot of physical tension. Writing shouldn't be such a big deal, should it? You're just sitting in a chair scribbling away, right? Next time you're in your regular writing space, pay attention to the way you're sitting, the way your fingers are poised over the keypad or wrapped around the pen. Notice your shoulders; creeping up toward your ears perhaps? Are you trying to hold up your arms with your shoulders or are you allowing the table to hold your weight? Is your jaw locked? Breath shallow? Brow furrowed? Shoulders hunched forward over the desk putting strain on your upper back? I'd bet all of you have noticed several, if not all, of these physical characteristics at some time while writing. You may even be exhibiting some of them now while you're reading. It seems as though we humans love to hold tension in our bodies. We have to retrain ourselves to move with freedom rather than contraction. To take the path of least effort rather than most effort when performing a simple physical activity. To use our breath like a bellows to keep our body expanding rather than contracting. To surrender rather than resist. When we consciously practice softening before we write, we've already taken a big step toward creating space and openness before we even pick up a pen. You can accomplish this softening in just a few breaths, or if you have the time on a particular morning, you can allow yourself fifteen minutes or more to pay attention to softening your body and mind.

Softening your body and mind is akin to stirring the raw ingredients in a cake mix. You can't make a cake until the batter is smooth. You want to have that same delicious buttery smoothness in your own body and breath. Earlier, when you opened your eyes and let your gaze caress the world around you, you were practicing "soft eyes." You weren't trying to see anything (attachment). You weren't trying not to see anything (aversion). This left space for you to see what you see. It gave you the space to practice absolute vulnerability without flinching.

Let's give a more practical example. If you go on a hike and try to see a hawk, your whole hiking experience will be measured against that intention. Did I see a hawk or didn't I? Maybe you do see a hawk, but you weren't able to get close enough to *really see* the hawk. You just saw it soaring across the sky. Does that count? Where does that fit in the story you constructed about your hike? By trying to see the hawk, you

Committing to Your Authentic Path

(consciously or unconsciously) filtered out things along the way that were not hawk. Maybe your gaze was focused only upward toward the sky or trees so you didn't see the small red flower pushing itself up through the roots of a ponderosa pine. Maybe you were focused on the trail map so you wouldn't get lost on your trek to find a hawk. When we're this focused, the likelihood of our seeing a hawk is miniscule, based solely on the chance that the hawk actually flies within the narrow window we've created for "hawk seeing."

This also applies to writing. When you're too narrowly focused on the intention of a book or a scene or a character, you close off possibilities that don't fit within the framework you've established.

This applies to self-knowledge as well. If you've boxed yourself in with labels and judgments, all the elements in the universe must conspire together perfectly for a sliver of authentic awareness to slip in.

The first part of the writing exercise in this chapter asked you to just observe your thoughts and write them down. This reinforced the softness, the flow, and the value of every aspect of your experience. Then I asked you to trust your intuition and choose a focal point to begin another piece of writing. This trained you to follow your own intuition and not seek outside direction for all your writing choices. However, instead of allowing you to wander off topic, I asked you to reign yourself back to the element you wanted to focus on. I asked you to do this a minimum of three times.

The two tasks weren't in opposition to each other, believe it or not. Writing is both flow and discipline. Art and craft. Intuition and perspiration. Writers have to create a lot of raw material to find the focus. A lot. Nobel Laureate and Holocaust survivor Elie Wiesel says, "There is a difference between a book of two hundred pages from the very beginning, and a book of two hundred pages which is the result of an original eight hundred pages. The six hundred are there. Only you don't see them." It's necessary to cultivate soft eyes to see those eight hundred pages. It's necessary to train your mind to discipline itself to stay on course so you can distill a clear, cohesive book of several hundred pages. Bringing your mind and your pen back to your original intention regularly helps cultivate that discipline. It also keeps you from moving away too quickly from something that might have a great deal of emotional energy for you. It's primal to move away from something painful. When we reach something in our writing that has an emotional charge, the sane thing to do is back away. The writer, however, can't look away. The writer stays, looks, absorbs, and reports. The writer's eyes stay clear and focused. That clarity and focus is grounded in softness, which is different from a focus that an outside source dictates to you. It's different from the kind that requires a rigid adherence to dogma. This focus comes authentically and organically from your direct experience. In yoga we talk about the importance of having strength *with* flexibility. Flexibility alone turns you into Gumby. Strength alone makes you a bulldozer.

In the beginning of this chapter, I referred to your body as your shell. Consider hermit crabs. They have a squishy and tender abdomen (just like us!), and they carry their shells on their backs as a home and as a barrier against the elements and predators. You've no doubt thought of your own body as a shell or container for your essence in some way or other. There's another layer of our human shell, though, and that's the energetic barrier we put up between others and ourselves. It's often much easier to soften our physical shell than our emotional and spiritual shells. I'm sure you've been in a situation where you've entered a room and noticed someone who absolutely positively not now not ever no how no way was going to let anyone into her personal sphere. She had a "keep out" wall in front of her wider than the span of the room. We can energetically feel that in others, and we respond by keeping our distance.

Hermit crabs use secondhand shells for their homes. They scavenge until they find a discarded shell, and then they move in. Think of the hermit crab's scavenged shell as similar to our own energetic shells. How much of your energetic shell—your barrier between your vulnerable, soft, squishy self and the rest of the world—is made up of ideas and belief systems that you've picked up secondhand? How much of it is not even yours, but scavenged from your parents, your ex-lovers, your tragic-poignant middle school experiences? How much of the rigidity, thickness, and depth of this energetic shell actually has anything at all to do with you? We tend to add bricks to our energetic wall when we get hurt. Hurt is real. Hurt sucks. Hurt also causes us to contract. The next time you bang your knee or accidentally cut your finger, try to relax into the pain rather than pull away from it. It's still going to hurt, but not as much. Promise. I've tried it. Hermit crabs know when their scavenged shells are no longer suitable. They leave the old shell in the sand and find a new home. Humans are a bit more stubborn. Rather than let things go as they arise, we're more likely to store them and then cover them with mortar to make sure they never move. Kind of maladaptive, don't you think?

In order to dive into our energetic walls so we can dismantle the bricks that aren't ours or no longer serve us, we have to cultivate a way of seeing these things that isn't going to magnify our resistance. This requires compassion, which is the final thing that soft eyes teach us. We learn first to turn compassion inward, so later we can authentically bring compassion into the world. We start by viewing ourselves with all our wrinkles and belly rolls and aching knees and mistakes without judgment. We leave space to look around honestly without fear and contraction. We then show ourselves that we can come to the table with clarity and compassion, not with the snarky schoolmarm or overbearing parent voice. Our authentic self takes notice, even if you don't notice yet. You're learning to cultivate intimacy with yourself. Once you've done that, you'll be able to extend that compassion into the world and into your writing.

CHAPTER 21

# Self-Study

Men can starve from a lack of self-realization as
much as they can from a lack of bread.

—Richard Wright

We have spent a good portion of this book engaged
in self-study, even if you haven't realized it. For
example, our shaking practice helps us pay more
attention to our inner and outer bodies. The Writing Warrior
practice pulls us back to our breath and to the page when we
want to stray. We're learning to sit and face our inner selves
without judgment. The more we uncover our authentic writing, the more we're uncovering ourselves.

Why is self-study important? Can't I write a best-selling
book without doing any of this inner work? Can't I do good
things in the world? Of course you can. But why would you
spend less time trying to understand yourself than you've
spent earning your degree or working on the craft of writing?
After all, you came in with you and you're going out with
you, nothing else. Wouldn't it be pretty cool if you knew who
that being was that you're traveling with?

In my experience, writers are natural questioners. This
might have gotten us in trouble in junior high, but it's a great

quality for someone wanting to explore the larger themes of the universe, or for someone who wants to solve the mystery of the clock tower, or understand more about black holes. Every book poses a question. Sometimes the writer is aware of this question in the beginning. Other times the question reveals itself as the writer writes. Part of the tension that keeps a reader wrapped up in a good book is a result of the reader wanting to know what happens next. The what, how, why, when, or where questions that propel a reader forward in a novel are the questions you use when exploring your own depths.

Last semester, a student said to me, "Laraine, I'm just not as deep as you think I am."

"Poppycock," I said.

We're all vast and limitless. What limits us is our patterns and our perceptions of what we think we can be. We likely have had some personal experience to support our claims, and that experience, rather than being a memory, becomes a taskmaster. Our responses today are often based on our experiences of yesterday. A guard to our inner depths has been trained to tell us there's nothing in there worth seeking, nothing in there worth exploring, and, most importantly, nothing in there worth loving. Over many years, we have learned to believe the guard is there even when he's taking a lunch break. We simply stop taking the trip.

It's frighteningly easy for our *habits* to become our facts, just like it's easy for our opinions of people, groups, and cultures to seem factual. But the warrior is ever vigilant. When your imaginary guard tells you to turn back, you stand your ground. "Why? Why should I turn back? You're not the boss of me!" And so you're able to take another step inward. Think of how many habits can become rigid assertions about ourselves over the course of our lives. A statement such as "I'm just not as deep as you think I am" becomes an unchallenged assumption. Unchallenged assumptions are the fuel that keeps the warrior from slaying dragons. For every unchallenged assumption in your mind, there are attached behaviors that may be harming yourself or others.

Psychoanalyst Carl Jung spent much of his life's work studying the unconscious self. It was his belief that the unconscious part of ourselves was what was really in charge of things, and that the more we could bring out of our unconscious to our conscious mind, the more harmonious our decisions and actions would be. We move into the unconscious first by the path of ruthless questioning. It's much easier to stay asleep. It's much easier to turn away when we're challenged with "poppycock" from an instructor.

It takes a great deal of energy to deny direct experience. Write that down. *It takes a great deal of energy to deny direct experience.* Why, then, do we not acknowledge the experience that's in front of us? We will have to experience it eventually because it is part of our path. When this student went back and looked at his writing and pushed further, he found he was able to uncover something, or at least bring forth something that he had buried for quite some time. He needed a push. We all need a push. Once something has arisen in our psyches, it's time to pay attention to it.

We've all got things buried. We have an abundance of experiences to uncover. I find that to be invigorating and exciting. What else can I look at? What else is keeping me from living my life as fully as I would like to? What else? What else? As you make more space within your body (please continue to do the shaking practice), you'll find images, memories, stories beginning to emerge, floating for a time and then passing away. Pay attention to these images. They are bread crumbs for you on your journey. Don't judge what comes up. Ideas such as, "Gosh, I can't believe I'm thinking about him again!" or "That's really too petty to be a problem" are examples of judging. It doesn't matter what comes up. If it comes up, it's yours. Own it.

What else? Walk right through the door to your inner depths to learn more. Once the guard there knows he can't push you away so easily, he'll back down. Now pay attention. This guard will get more clever the more work you do, and he'll find ways to trick you into turning away again. Be ever vigilant. Question everything. Don't be complacent. When something that arises feels right, embrace it. If a time comes when that belief or concept no longer feels authentic to you, let it go. It's easy to embrace what feels right, often not so easy to let it go later. Remember this Taoist wisdom: When the guest comes, make hot tea. When the guest leaves, throw it out. In other words, welcome what arises in the moment. Don't attach. Don't avert. When what arises passes, don't hold on.

Self-study requires mindful courage. It requires you to stand steady when you're confronted with your own patterns and responses. It requires you to look through your initial reactions until you see their tender root at your center. When you are able to look with soft eyes, it's easier for self-judgments to fall away. It requires great courage to remain steady while gazing into one's own eyes. It takes great will to keep your gaze steady as you continue to open and open and open into absolute vulnerability.

Filmmaker Akira Kurosawa says, "To be an artist means to never avert your eyes." Keep looking. Especially when you want to turn away. By standing steady, you'll learn something new. And here's the really cool part—when you learn something new, you can let something old go. Cast off what does not serve you.

Drop it.

Plink. Plink.

Into the red bucket.

There is no sorrow from the tree as it sheds its leaves. No sorrow from the clouds as they release their rain. Take the red bucket and scatter its contents to the wind. Nothing in nature is waste. What no longer serves you will sustain another.

Bow to what you cast away and rise each day lighter.

## CHAPTER 22

# Wake Up

Self-observation brings man to the realization of the necessity of self-change. And in observing himself a man notices that self-observation itself brings about certain changes in his inner processes. He begins to understand that self-observation is an instrument of self-change, a means of awakening.

—George Gurdjieff

Keep the blinds drawn! Stay snug and warm under your down comforter. Ignore the footsteps you hear downstairs. Ignore the tapping of the branches on your windows. Turn the clock away from you so you cannot see its amber glow in the darkness. How many more hours do you have left until you must rise?

I don't know about you, but one of my all-time favorite features on an alarm clock is the snooze button. I set the alarm for an hour before I actually need to get up so I can press the snooze button six times. After six times, I know it's time to really wake up, no more time for lingering in the soft and squishy place of not quite sleep, not quite awake. This is a seductive place. I often feel like there are literal weights on my body, keeping me in bed longer than I should be. Pushing through those weights requires great willpower on some days. I feel like I'm swimming through warm honey, trying to break through the surface into the daylight.

I feel as though I spend most of my life in this between-sleep-and-awake space. I get lazy and want to just stay asleep. It's easier. Requires no action. No warrior poses. No staring at my illusions and delusions, trying to slay them with the proverbial sword of enlightenment. Just sleeping, oh so comfortably, until something painful wakes me up. I've observed that the universe is pretty fast and furious when it comes to sending something painful to wake me up. I try now to pay attention to the first mosquito bite, rather than waiting for a ravenous tiger to leap into my life and turn everything upside down.

It's easy to get stuck in the half-sleep/half-awake space. We're busy. We're in our cars a lot. We're commuting from one place to another. We're worried about our jobs, our families, our health care, and our planet's health. We are taking care of aging parents or special-needs children. We are working several jobs and going to night school. We are campaigning. Organizing. Volunteering. Sometimes I catch myself midsleep and notice that I've done an awful lot on a particular day, but I have no clear memory of any of it. I sometimes notice when I'm driving that I somehow end up getting off at the right exit, but I don't always remember how I got there or what was going on at the exits along my route. I've often joked about trying to figure out what part of me is paying attention when most of me seems to be asleep. Who was driving that car while I was remembering a trip to Virginia in 1980? Too scary to think about. I shake my head. Wake up, Laraine! Pay attention!

Times like the ones I just described are times when the mind has moved into the past or future, often into a place of anxiety over what could happen later that day or week, or what happened earlier in the day or many years ago. The mind has checked out and gone to a story line it's comfortable with. It doesn't want to pay attention to driving (or waiting in the doctor's office, or reading, or taking a walk). It wants to be someplace else—not because I'm a bad person who doesn't want to wake up, but because *that's what the mind does.* Oh! There you go again! Gotcha! Come on back to now. And then, in the microsecond it takes for our mind to go wandering off again—gotcha! Come on back to now. And over and over and over. Your breathing practice helps to discipline your mind to catch itself. The soft eyes writing practice helps to reign in your mind. Learning to return to the page to follow the next right word rather than worrying about what you're going to do in chapter seven helps your mind learn to catch itself. You'll never still your mind. But you can watch it, and in the watching, you'll find yourself changing.

The Writing Warrior cannot remain complacent. You cannot sleepwalk through your life. You cannot tune out your characters' voices, the questions that pull at you in the middle of the night, the images you cannot erase. The Writing Warrior sets the alarm, gets up, and pays attention because there is no other option. You know that to turn your back on what you see is a betrayal of your writing.

During my yoga teacher training program, my teacher taught us the importance of not telling people in a yoga class to change their personal habits or behaviors. He didn't want us to be attached to people's behaviors—eating meat, not eating meat, drinking or not drinking caffeine or alcohol, smoking or not smoking; whatever a yogi is "supposed" to do didn't matter. Through practice and through paying attention, habits and behaviors that no longer serve the individual will eventually fall away.

Wake up. The more you notice, the more you notice. And the more you notice, the fewer obstacles will block your path.

## CHAPTER 23

# Perhaps You Never Did This, But I Remember It Just the Same

A memory is what is left when something happens and does not completely unhappen.

—Edward de Bono

O nce upon a time, a little girl and a little boy went to the playground to ride the seesaw. The little girl had brown hair and wore a pink fluffy snowsuit. The little boy wore a green fleece jacket and had one brown mitten and one blue mitten. The day was clear, though snow had just fallen the night before. The little girl and little boy were proud to be old enough to go to the park by themselves, now that they'd reached the very old ages of eight and ten.

"Remember?" said the little girl, now thirty-one, now never wearing pink. "Remember that day we got to go to the park by ourselves and you fell off the seesaw and tore your blue jacket?"

"I remember the park," said the little boy, now thirty-three. "But it wasn't me who fell off. It was you. And I never had a blue jacket. You always remember colors wrong. My jacket was red. Chicago Bulls red."

I'll bet you've all had a conversation like this one. This is a pretty benign event though, right? Kids fall down. Does it really matter if the jacket was blue, green, or red? Probably not. But what if this day was more significant than that? What if this was the day when a flash flood came through town, or a tornado, or what if it was the day when they found out their parents were getting a divorce? What if the little boy had been kidnapped that day, and all the little girl had was her memory of the jacket to tell the law enforcement officers who were trying to find her brother? What if, what if—the stuff of stories. Writers love the "what if" question. It sets us off on wild plot chases and wilder character interactions. Whenever we get stuck in a chapter, we can play the "what if" game and keep writing for a little while longer.

Memory is much more like art than science. Memory is not absolute. Memory has shadows and stories, just as individual words do. Just as "playground" doesn't conjure up the same image for everyone, each person present at a particular event will remember different things. What we remember is not based on a formula, but rather is a montage, or collage, of events that made it through our filter as somehow significant. This happens through triggers—things we're attached to, things we're repulsed by, and things we're attracted to. If a song on the radio is an old Elvis tune, I might retain that memory because my dad loved Elvis and he's dead and I miss him, so the Elvis song carries some significance for me. Maybe the song playing was "Blue Suede Shoes," but after a few days I remember it as "You Ain't Nothin' but a Hound Dog" because that's my own favorite Elvis song. Memory layers itself upon itself. It forms its own Gordian knot, which not only gets repeated over time as we "remember," but shifts as we have more experiences and impressions and understandings about a particular event. Memories become colored by what our hopes and desires were for that particular experience, and by the effect that experience has had on us throughout our lives. Our memories also become colored by others who shared that experience with us.

When working with memory in your writing (and you are, whether you're writing fiction, memoir, or poetry), understand that you're working with not *what happened* but rather your *perception* of what happened. This is a very important distinction. Writers get worked up over the notion of truth and memory. Here's the deal. Memory may never be "truth" as it relates to a specific sequence of events. What memory can be is an essential truth for you—an authentic expression of an emotional experience, rather than a literal experience. Here's the rest of the deal—it doesn't necessarily matter if you no longer know what really happened. What matters when you first begin the warrior work of self-study is what you believe happened. *That* story is currently affecting you. It doesn't matter if it never happened in "real" life. If you believe it happened, then for our purposes, and for the purposes of how your body holds emotions and experiences, it did happen. Just accept that. Listen to your body as well as your memory as you try to figure out what makes you tick and why.

Amy Tan says, "I have a writer's memory which makes everything worse than maybe it actually was." Because I've always adored story, and because I have always been resistant to change, I've spent a great deal of time hanging out in the frozen halls of memory. Working and reworking a memory until I'm truly no longer sure what happened or, sometimes, if it even happened at all. For me, remembering seems to take me further and further away from the *actual* event and closer to one of the following two options: what I'd have liked to have happened or the way the event has affected me. I instinctively want to arrange a series of events so it will have the biggest dramatic impact on me and my readers (listeners, friends, family). Life doesn't always happen in the appropriate order to have the greatest dramatic effect on people. Also, if I unconsciously want to remain attached to a particular story line or belief system about a person, I can rearrange the events, and then stress the situation's unpleasantness or pleasantness to suit my objective.

We exaggerate our stories without thinking about it when we're not paying attention. It's natural to want to be seen in the best light, to want people to love and respect us, to have a place to belong with friends and family. It takes a great deal of risk to not always be the star of your memory story. For true ruthless self-study, you must be willing to entertain the possibility that you're not always doing everything right, or, if you tend to believe you are always messing everything up, you have to be willing to consider that you might actually not be the worst person in the universe after all.

Over many years, we exaggerate, reform, and erase our memories to build a story we live by as gospel truth. Holidays mesh together until you can't remember whether it was Thanksgiving 1964 or Christmas 1978 when Uncle Frank threw the whiskey bottle across the room and smashed the vase your great-grandmother had brought all the way from Finland when she immigrated to the United States in 1924. Maybe it wasn't even a whiskey bottle. Maybe it wasn't even Uncle Frank. Maybe it was your father, and you don't want to remember because your father's been dead for ten years now and you really don't want to think about anything he might have done that was less than upstanding.

We have to accept our memories with a grain of salt. Don't worry that your memories aren't always accurate. The awareness that they aren't will help you see things more clearly. Part of what we're working with here is our human desire to always be right. If you believe it was Uncle Frank who threw the vase and your relationship with Uncle Frank has been strained ever since, then what matters in your own development is what you believe happened. Your next step in ruthless self-study is to question. Are you sure? Why are you sure? Is there corroborating evidence? Is there anyone else who can substantiate your story? You're the one who's being affected by your interpretation of events. Keep that first and foremost in mind. Then hold to the possibility that your interpretations have been shaped by your unconscious desires. What story have you told yourself about your life that you might be willing to let go of?

I worked diligently on my autobiography from kindergarten through the summer of my seventh year. I had two volumes going by the time summer 1976 rolled around. Part 1 was called *My Name Is Laraine* and featured a colored-pencil drawing of my sister and me holding hands (something I can never remember us doing) and skipping down the street. It had chapters like "John Walker" (my first crush) and "Peanut Butter Cookies" (the snack we had in kindergarten one day).

Part 2 was called, appropriately, *More My Name Is Laraine*. Part 2 was mostly an outline for chapters to come, but part 1 had a narrative, which was accurate enough to help me remember that I had a frog cubbyhole in kindergarten to put my things in, and that I made a macaroni Christmas tree for my mother out of a toilet paper roll in first grade. I had assigned, in pencil on the cover's upper-right corner, a price of $1.50 for each book. My dedication and acknowledgments page went on far too long. I was six and already thanking everyone I'd ever met for helping me with my story. I knew instinctively that no one's story exists alone.

I worked on those books with devotion and ease. I wrote in my bedroom, with a blue No. 2 pencil. I was careful not to press too hard on the paper because I was certain that once the pencil reached the nub stage of its life, I'd have no more words. I always wrote with my door closed, facing a pink wall. I wrote dialogue and description, loving the quotation marks that to me indicated not just what someone had said, but what I had *heard*. It didn't occur to me then that those might not be the same thing.

I bore witness to my life and all its minor scenes (the death of Gus, the black bubble-eyed goldfish; the visit to Daddy's office where there were rows and rows of—*imagine the joy*—typewriters; scooping lima beans off my plate into my lap and then running to the bathroom to dump them in the toilet, starving African children be damned). I was sure, without anyone ever telling me, that it mattered to keep a record of my stories.

I wasn't thinking yet about organization or structure or style. I was just selecting events that seemed the most meaningful and then recording them on the page. Not a whole lot of reflection occurred, beyond the "it was fun" or "it was yucky" type, but a foundation for a writer's eye emerged. I have kept these volumes, along with boxes of diaries and journals, all my life. I cannot imagine throwing them out, even though I almost never look at them. When I do visit them, I don't recognize myself, which I guess is an essential understanding for a memoirist. The "I" I am now is not the "I" who lived then. The "I" writing this will not exist in one more second.

In 2004, when I moved from Phoenix to Prescott, Arizona, at thirty-six years old, I looked back at my autobiographies. In previous glances, I'd been secretly proud of my ability to punctuate dialogue correctly at six, pleased as punch that I spelled almost every word right and that I used subordinating clauses naturally. This time, I saw where the narrative stopped—sometime in late July 1976.

I had a red-and-green diary from the fifth grade, 1978, but nothing from summer of 1976 until then. I had stopped. Where did the story go if it wasn't put on the page? Where did the experiences move to? What exactly happened? The last chapter in my autobiography is called "Daddy Had a Heart Attack."

*One Sunday in August of 1976, Melanie rushed into Laraine's bedroom, shouting, "Daddy had a heart attack! Daddy had a heart attack!" And she jumped all over her.*

*When she got off, Laraine said, "Liar."*

*"You want to bet?" Melanie said. "Vicki and Frederick are coming to stay with us while Mama goes to the hospital to visit."*

*"Oh." Laraine got up to see if Melanie was telling the truth. She was. Vicki and Frederick had just walked in the back door. "Oh no!" Laraine started screaming at God and then burst into tears. Vicki came over to see if she could help. But nobody could. Not even Mama.*

And that was the end of my autobiography. I wish that, instead of knowing that end punctuation goes inside quotation marks, I'd known what happens to writers when they stop writing their stories. But if I had known that then, I wouldn't have a story to tell you now, so as they say, it all works out for the best.

When I think about those weeks after Dad's heart attack, I honestly can't be sure what I remember and what I've been told happened. I don't think anymore that it matters which is which. I think what's more striking is my absence of emotions connected to the events at the time.

James Pennebaker, one of the early researchers in writing as a healing tool, wrote of the importance not just of recording the events, but also of reflecting on them and expressing feelings around them. Nowhere in my childhood autobiography chapter did I express a single feeling word. Nowhere did I reflect on the meaning of the events or on what I thought the larger impact of the events would be. This is perhaps not unusual, given that I was seven, but that, combined with the cease and desist order I apparently gave my writing mojo, assures me that this stopping of my narrative is extremely important in some way.

We write from memory, whether event-based or emotion-based. We empathize with the abused child in our novel because we remember a time when someone hurt us. Our memories shape our worldview. They help formulate the questions we deem valuable and worth exploring. They are the things that haunt us and draw us to the page.

Let me try and remember now.

I remember the forest green carpet of our living room, dining room, and hallway. I remember dime-store paintings of hunting dogs on our fake wood-paneled den walls. I remember the curlicue pattern of the beige-and-black tile (linoleum?) in the kitchen and den. Our sofa was also green, and, in only eleven short years, it would become my first sofa in my first apartment. The sliding glass door had thick gold drapes with a white rubber backing. The piano was in the dining room, which was never used to eat in, only used for storing things— cool things like my train set and my red car, big enough for a whole person to sit in and ride! The dining room was my mother's junk room, the need for which is a genetic defect that I have also inherited. I remember a Wiffle ball and a red plastic baseball bat. A beige rotary phone that hung on the wall beside the side door. Orange, brown, and gold curtains my mother made for the kitchen windows. She'd stand at the sink washing dishes and look out into the front yard and watch me playing with my best friend, Donna, or watch me sitting by the sewers at the foot of our steep hill yard, wondering where all the water went.

The morning my dad had a heart attack, someone else's perfume was in the house. That morning, we should have been going to church. There should have been bacon and egg smells, and coffee should have burped in the stovetop perco-lator. That morning should have been—wait. Stop. I'm try-ing too hard. I'm trying to put together the elements I think should be there. But they're not there. What do I remember? Perhaps a better question: what do I feel? I feel a key to a lock I didn't know I had. I feel a slamming of doors, which still reverberate in my belly. I feel a change coming (ah, narrative, the moment of change occurs when . . .), but not that kind of change. I feel sideswiped by this change, this change I didn't know could possibly happen.

I cry out to the leader of my story, Jesus, and hear nothing. My story line is failing. My daddy is gone and the house is so very very big. Uncertainty hangs from the rubber-backed drapes. Leftover food from last night's dinner is still in the refrigerator. Another woman's perfume is in the house. My mother's friend Vicki is here to take us to Bob's Big Boy and then swimming. My mother's friend Vicki is not my mother. She is not my father. She doesn't even know how to make scrambled eggs right. They're too hard and dry, and she put pepper on them without asking. The sun is coming up like any other day. The same sun that yesterday bathed me in its grace as I swung on my yellow swing. This sun is too bright, too light, too aggressive. How dare it shine in my window on this day when everything changed?

No . . . here's what I remember:

The chair my dad sat in that July night in 1976 to eat his dish of chocolate ice cream was a slick, brown vinyl La-Z-Boy. When he reclined, it snapped back into place with the emphasis of an exclamation point. *Chico and the Man* and *Sanford and Son* were on the television. Dinner had been steak and french fries, hamburgers for my sister and me, ice cream for all of us. Our Charlotte, North Carolina, neighbor-hood was quiet by 8:30 AM that night. The air conditioner blew icy air to dilute the heat and humidity. My black, bubble-eyed goldfish named Gus swam in circles above red and blue rocks. Nothing ever changed for Gus until the day he turned over on his side and went away.

I liked to go to bed when Mama and Daddy were still talking. The television's artificial sounds and my mother's soprano laughter were underscored by my father's baritone, so deep and low that sometimes I couldn't decipher his words. The tones became a tune—bass clef, treble clef—conducting the symphony of my dreams.

That night I never heard a sound. I slept in my four-poster bed under a frilly pink canopy decorated with Victorian-style ladies carrying parasols, eternally dancing. My bookcase made of two-by-fours and bricks never even creaked a warning during the night. Even my precious stories had let me down.

Eight o'clock in the morning. The sun cut squares through the window; the house was way too quiet. I didn't smell bacon or eggs or coffee. Mama should have woken me up by now. I walked down the hall, dragging my security blanket over olive green shag carpet. A woman, my mother's friend Vicki, sat in my father's chair. She looked small in it, like a child wearing dress-up clothes. The TV flashed Captain Kangaroo and Mr. Green Jeans, but the sound was off. Vicki saw me, ground out her cigarette, and said, "You're going to have to be strong now." And she opened her arms to me and I went to her, eyes still full of sleep, but when she wrapped her tanned, bare arms around my shoulders, she didn't smell like Mama, and breakfast wasn't ready, and Vicki drank tea instead of coffee, and I thought I saw something black—a rider on horseback—in the corner of the den. "Your father had a heart attack. Your mother is with him now. You and your sister are coming to stay with me. We'll get Bob's Big Boy and then go to the pool. Won't that be fun?"

The dark rider in the corner of the room waited. His horse shifted its weight. Death had come for my father. Now it was waiting to see what I would do. Where was sweet Jesus with his swift and powerful sword? Where was his love? What if Daddy didn't really believe in the secret places of his heart that Jesus was the son of God? If he didn't believe, God would know and Daddy would go to hell. I started to cry, not because I understood what death could mean for me, but because I feared the suffering death could mean for Daddy. How could I ever know if he was OK? How could I ever know that God had welcomed him?

"Do you want to pray?" asked Vicki. I shook my head. Whatever was going to happen was done. Praying could do no good. Vicki tried to hold me again. "It's all right. God understands." I pulled away from her and went to the piano. I'd been taking lessons for a year. I tried to play "Amazing Grace" like Daddy would play it, but I couldn't. All the notes were right, but when I put them all together, the tune danced away from me, laughing at my faith that simply reading the music properly could make the song sound beautiful.

Daddy didn't die that day. He came home from the hospital after many weeks. He stayed in bed. I went to the third grade and learned about asteroids and verbs. The bicentennial celebration was over. The flags and the dresses and the red, white, and blue Jell-O molds disappeared, so slowly you hardly noticed—like Daddy. Like Jesus.

Here's what I know:

That night I never heard a sound. I slept in my four-poster bed under a frilly pink canopy decorated with Victorian-style ladies carrying parasols, eternally dancing. My bookcase made of two-by-fours and bricks never even creaked a warning during the night. Even my precious stories had let me down.

Memory. The stuff of hopes and hauntings. Everything a Writing Warrior will ever need.

CHAPTER 24

# Stories We Tell Ourselves

Reality is merely an illusion, although a very persistent one.

—Albert Einstein

I celebrated my eighth birthday during the few weeks my sister and I spent in Wilmington when Dad was in the hospital. My grandparents and aunt and uncle had given me a party complete with homemade chocolate cake and chocolate ice cream. Grandma gave me a model of the *Santa Maria*. "One day you can have the other two ships," she said. That seemed amazing to me, owning the three ships that sailed to America, even if they were fakes. "You know, the Herring family was one of the first to settle in North Carolina. We go back to the sixteen hundreds." I knew Grandma went back to 1909, which was ancient enough. "We're an old family. Don't let anyone tell you any different. We belong here." I didn't know what "we belong here" meant, but when she died in 1996 and willed the cornfield to my sister and me with precise instructions not to sell the land to anyone outside the family, I was pretty sure what weight those words carried. We belong here. Masonboro Sound. North Carolina.

The creek and the field and the woods. The alligator and the quail and the mosquitoes.

After we moved to Arizona, I would play John Denver's "Country Roads" over and over again until I believed I could look out my window in the Phoenix desert and see weeping willows and thick dragonflies with wings the colors of crystals. It never worked. But I kept hoping. Hoping that back to school would again mean sweaters and mittens held together with a single piece of yarn. It didn't occur to me that I was not looking for a place—not a house, not Springfield Drive, not Idlewild Elementary School—but for a time when I was someone else.

When I think now about returning to North Carolina, I think first about the stories I've told myself about it. I think about the scents from bushels of flowers too numerous to name hanging around me like vats of expensive perfume. I'm afraid, yet pulled into the open green doors of an African American Baptist church where the ladies still wear white gloves and tall pink hats and sing on cue from a place I try to reach with words, but always fall one or two notes short.

I think of sweet tea and of tomatoes that leave no doubt in my mind that they are a fruit. I think of dinner on the grounds and little white church after little white church lined up along state rural routes like daisies. I think of porches with three cement steps leading up to them and lean-to shacks left over from a different Southern story line.

When I think about going back, I want to take only the route that will lead through my stories. I don't want my story to butt up against three decades of changes. I want Mrs. Whisenhunt to still be teaching second grade at Idlewild Elementary School. I want to be able to walk into room 203 and see my seven-year-old self reading a book in one of the blue plastic chairs. I want to sit down with her and look out the open window (but surely the school is air conditioned by now?) onto the school's front lawn, where I learned to fly a kite on a March day that was too warm for winter and too cold for spring. I want to see the cursive alphabet, each letter on a bright yellow rectangle, dancing atop a black chalkboard.

My spelling book is maroon with a gold 2 on the cover. I am the best speller in the class. So good, in fact, that when I get to fifth grade I go to the state spelling bee where I lose in the final round with the word *sukiyaki*. What self-respecting Southerner in 1978 had eaten sukiyaki? To this day, I am hard pressed to eat Japanese food. I wanted to go to the White House and meet Jimmy Carter, who seemed to me incredibly nice and sensible. I had heard he was a poet too, and that made him special. Instead, we went to Columbus, Georgia, to visit the people who came to stay with my sister and me the night Dad had his heart attack.

I want the houses to all be painted the colors I remember—our brick house still sporting red shutters and beige doors, my best friend Donna's house still yellow and brown, still the house it was before it caught on fire. I want Tony, the old bulldog from next door, to bark and growl at every rustle of leaves on the other side of the chain link fence, the friendly fence before they built the solid wood one to separate our two houses after we sold our home to a black couple in 1981. I want the dark brown butter churn my grandmother gave us to be outside by the storeroom, still a warm bed for Charley, the black tomcat. I want Ron to be driving the school bus my sister and I took to school, stopping right at our driveway so we could run inside and grab a Little Debbie snack cake for him. I want there to still be the possibility that Jesus will come and save us, wrapped in a honey-baked ham and sweet potato pie.

I want to step into an open picture book that I've left untouched beside the bed for thirty years. I want everything to be the same—maybe a little faded—but essentially the same. I want the apple tree we planted in the backyard where we buried a school of goldfish to be only a sapling. I want to not yet know how to do long division or conjugate Latin verbs or bury a father. I want to sit down at the particleboard dining room table with the leaf in and hold hands with everyone who isn't here anymore, pass a plate of Carolina pulled BBQ pork (it's the vinegar that makes the difference) and a bowl of collard greens cooked all day long, lift our glasses of sweet tea, and bow our heads to the Baby Jesus, who, one by one, took us all away.

But home is not a place. It is a person I used to be, and because of that, and because it is true you can't step in the same river twice, home's become a shadow, something I catch out of the corner of my eye but can't quite touch because she, the person I used to be, is inside me.

What stories do you tell yourself about home? Family? Love? Relationships? Money? Fame? Success? Understanding these stories will help you understand yourself. You'll notice that your stories about things continue to surface in your stories and poems. One function of literature is to help illuminate the dark and light places within us. But there's another function too. Literature can help us release the stories that don't serve us anymore, and writing will transform you, if you're enough of a warrior to let it.

Your stories about yourself, whether about home, family, or missed opportunities, are nestled in your bones. They inform your choices and they create your limitations. Each time you write your story, you move it. It becomes a little less solidified, a little more fluid. Each time you put pen to paper, you revise your story, releasing a little bit, reconstructing a little bit, looking at yourself through the lens of yourself today. Each time you write your story, you make more room in your physical and emotional bodies. When you know what stories you're carrying, you're less likely to make present choices based on past experience. You're less likely to avoid potential experiences based on past fears and disappointments. As you do your shaking practice, you are also making room. You are breaking up physical stagnation. You're releasing stories. And in this way, the Writing Warrior, with each stroke of the pen, stands a bit more free.

## CHAPTER 25

# Revision

If you're really listening, if you're awake to the
poignant beauty of the world, your heart breaks
    regularly.
In fact, your heart is made to break;
its purpose is to burst open again and again
so that it can hold ever-more wonders.

—Andrew Harvey

ew things strike fear in the hearts of writers more
than the notion of revision. I'm not sure if it's laziness
(trying to avoid the work of fine-tuning and reshaping your work), self-loathing (if I didn't get it right the first
time I'm just not a writer anyway), an unwillingness to work
at the nuts and bolts of the craft, a reluctance to look at the
internal issues or questions that pulled the story out of you
in the first place, a strange arrogance that you are somehow
brilliant enough to have "gotten it right" the first time, or
some combination of all these things. I want to address revision both in terms of your development as a person who
writes and within the realm of the craft.

John Irving says, "There's no reason you shouldn't, as a
writer, not be aware of the necessity to revise yourself con-

stantly." This is an interesting approach to the writer's work. Have you ever fallen in love with an author, only to discover that he or she keeps writing the same book over and over again, whether conceptually, thematically, or structurally? By the time you read their fifth book, you know exactly what epiphanies the protagonist will have and what flaws the antagonist will have. You'll likely find yourself bored with the story and with the writer. It can be easy to mine the same field over and over again.

However, it can be especially challenging when a writer is lucky enough to have found success in a particular genre. Publishers tend to want more of the same type of work that already sold well. This is a blessing and a curse. Yay for wanting more of your writing! Sigh for being unable to stretch and grow as an artist as far as you feel drawn to grow. You might notice it in actors as well; the guy who gets typecast as a deadbeat dad seems to always show up as a deadbeat dad. Tried and true. As an artist, you must be ever-vigilant when it comes to pushing yourself forward in your craft. You must resist the call of the familiar (and believe me, it's a seductive call). You must resist the call of predictability and acceptability and push yourself deeper into your own work.

Revision begins with relentlessly questioning yourself and your work. What are you doing that you've already done before? Is there a way you can do it differently? Better? Deeper? Do you have anything left to say about that idea or those characters? Where can you go in your work that feels unfamiliar? A little scary, even? Those are places to move into more deeply. Those are places to pay attention to. Don't let your work get stale; the surest way to avoid that pitfall is to keep changing yourself. Don't let stagnation, patterning, and familiarity become your deepest companions. It's frighteningly easy to do. They feel like old friends.

Revising yourself involves the same steps as revising

your work. You have to be ruthlessly honest. You have to be willing to look at yourself with soft eyes and compassion. You have to be willing to ask the tough questions: Is this behavior serving me or is it time to let it go? Is this the real issue I'm dealing with or is there something underneath it? Something I've been avoiding? As you learn to trust yourself, you'll find changes happening without effort. As you practice surrender rather than resistance, you'll find those changes less stressful and painful. Watch yourself without judgment. Pay attention. Prune away what is choking you so what's underneath can bloom.

When it comes to the craft of writing, some writers handle the big *R* word better than others, but students who are new to creative writing, and new to writing as a process rather than a product, often have a difficult time handling the idea and stages of revision. You all know the cliché: real writers revise. It's one of those clichés that's a cliché because it's true. But revision in creative writing isn't like it was for your English classes. You don't just go in and do what the teacher said to do in her red ink and call it a day. That's lazy at its best, disrespectful to your work at its worst.

Nothing begins to break down the sneaky edges of the ego like the writing process. Let it happen. Let yourself be opened over and over again, as far and as deep and as wide as you can go. Here are some thoughts on revision that may be helpful.

1. Accept that you cannot see your work clearly. All writers should have "readers"—friends in a writing group, colleagues, agents, and so on—and we need them like we need oxygen. The more you write and the more you read, the better you'll be able to see your work, but there will always be blind spots because you're looking at it through your own beautifully tinted eyeballs.

2. Accept the necessary detachment from your work. Just because you wrote it doesn't make it precious or priceless or perfect. You just wrote it. Let that be enough. Over time and practice, you may come to believe that the fact that you wrote it really is enough, and that is far more than you thought it could be. No good, no bad, just what it is. Everything you write—everything—brings you closer to the next place. No words are wasted. No attempts are worthless. You wrote it. It is that, and nothing more. Yet see how that is everything?

3. Think of writing early drafts (like, say, the first five or so) as scattering seeds. You throw a handful of seeds into a hole in the earth and you wait. You don't really know what you put in the ground yet. You don't know what will be able to grow compatibly, or what will have to be pruned out and planted somewhere else. You've got to let things grow a bit before you can see what's up.

4. Hard part here: WAIT. Imagine some buffed-up cop (or maybe Johnny Depp) saying, "Back away from the manuscript, ma'am. Just back away now!" To go back to my seed analogy, what happens after you throw the seeds into the earth? You've got to water them and then wait. Sometimes we have to wait two whole seasons to see what pops out of the ground. I'm currently going back to a project I wrote seven years ago. The time for it is now. Yeah, really, writing is like that.

5. After you wait a while, read your work again. Not with an eye for tearing it apart, but with an ear for listening with compassion to what you were trying to say. One of my favorite teachers told me to use "teabag listening." He was talking about letting the tea steep for a while and then, over time, listening to (tasting) what flavors surfaced. Be gentle here. Don't be manic with your work or with yourself. Let your work speak to you while you turn off your critic/editor/ shame-based voice (whatever your baggage is from other

classes or groups or family) and nod and say thank-you. Don't listen to your work with a knife at its throat. How much do you think it'll actually say to you that way?

6. Observe what you've sown. If you've listened well and authentically, you might now notice that you threw seeds for a pine tree, a strawberry plant, and a sunflower in the same hole. What are the odds that all three story arcs can coexist in the same hole in the ground? Pretty slim. So which story is fighting for survival? Which one desperately wants you to hear it? I don't know the answer for any individual, but I know a key to finding out is to ask this question: which one did I not know was there? You might do well to remember that the plant (yes, I'm going to extend this metaphor all the way through) that is bullying the other plants may not be the one you really need to write about. The loudest isn't always the most powerful.

7. Start again. Yes. Again. Dig a new hole (clean piece of paper, empty computer file) and scatter a different handful of seeds again. Maybe this time·75 percent of them are sunflower seeds and only a few are oak trees or eggplants. Wait some more. Maybe you'll wait as long as the last time, maybe not. But wait. Let things settle and integrate and assemble without you constantly hacking at the roots.

8. What blooms now?

Get the picture? All throughout this process, you're reading. You're still writing too. There's no rule that says thou must only work on one thing at a time. You're reading, and, did I mention, you're reading?

Revision teaches you a lot about yourself. I encourage you as you begin your revisions to observe your own behavior. Observe it with the same non-knife-wielding compassion that you use while listening to your work. Notice something, and say, "Hmmm. Look at that." If it's not working for you, stop doing it. But don't shame yourself about it. We're all beautifully flawed. If you're tearing yourself up inside and causing suffering to yourself, stop. Ask yourself why you're causing yourself pain. The answer might surprise you. Over time, you'll clear out your gut-wrenching resistances to revision, and you'll find absolute freedom and joy in re-envisioning a piece of your writing. You'll know that you can toss out those pages because more will come. You'll know that nothing is wasted. But it takes time to know these things in your body, and if you're doing this for the first time, expect some suffering. I offer these things to you in the hopes that you can shorten your period of suffering and move more quickly into the freedom of the process. We as writers can resist this stage or we can embrace it. The act itself (the revision) is neutral. Our reaction to it shapes everything.

Revision teaches a lot, indeed. But the biggest thing it will teach you is: are you a writer? And if it turns out you're not, no big deal. There are lots of glorious things to do in this world that don't involve so much solitude and ink. Approach everything with openness. Where there's resistance, there's struggle. Where there's struggle, there's conflict. Go back to that voice I mentioned earlier that's compelling you to put something on paper. What does it have to tell you? My guess is that it's saying you're a writer.

And if all this falls short, remember these words from Margaret Atwood: "A ratio of failures is built into the process of writing. The wastebasket has evolved for a reason."

CHAPTER 26

# Intuition

Trust thyself. Every heart vibrates to that iron
string.

—Ralph Waldo Emerson

B elieve it or not, there was a time when you knew
the next right thing to do. Some of you might even
remember when that time was, or a circumstance
where you trusted your intuition. For a lot of us, though,
our intuition was one of the things that got pushed out of
our psyches in favor of concrete data and proven formulas
for actions and responses. It's our intuition that tells us not
to walk down that particular street even though there's no
rational reason not to. It's our intuition that chooses the
cobalt blue crayon to paint the horse's mane with, even as
our logical mind tells us that horses' manes aren't cobalt
blue. It's our intuition that calls us to a particular teacher's
writing class, or a class in weaving, or invites us to stop in at
the corner café on the day the man you're going to marry will
walk in. It's our intuition that tells us when it's time to end
a relationship (even though it may take our rational minds
years to take action on this). It's our intuition that helps us
choose the puppy from the pound to take home or pull the

book off the bookshelf that's just right for what's going on in your life.

It's also your intuition that drops a character you've never imagined smack dab in the middle of your novel and demands that you investigate her. Sometimes this intuition is a trickster. Sometimes this intuition brings you the deepest synchronicity in your work. You won't know its gifts until you follow it along the path.

Don't reject your intuition because your rational mind tells you something else. Don't have a preconceived idea in mind for a story that shuts out the surprises that inevitably surface along any writer's path. Don't stomp your feet and cry, "No! No! Not in my story! Not in this poem!" Back away. Listen.

As you may have already ascertained, trusting one's intuition involves trusting one's self, making space, and developing a relationship with your own inner teacher. If you fundamentally don't believe that you have anything of value to tell yourself (watch this closely; you may not be aware that you believe this, but your actions and reactions demonstrate a lack of trust in yourself), then you will always be in a place of chasing outer validation. It's risky to use your intuition to carry a novel through a first draft. After all, most of us have been well-schooled in how to make action plans and mission statements. We learned how to navigate the school system with its multiple-choice assessment tests and quantitative objectives.

Intuition is the magic in the writing process. The magic doesn't come from the mountaintop. It doesn't come from your finicky, persnickety muse who comes and goes with the wind. It doesn't come in the form of a lightning bolt or a thunderclap. The magic comes from that still small voice within you that may be only a whisper right now, but it's there. Listen. Listen. Find the way back to that voice, and as it recognizes your commitment to trusting it, it will become louder. Before you know it, you'll rely first on intuition, next on hard cold data. Allow the relationship between you and your intuition to flourish by staying in open communication with it.

All the tools we're cultivating will strengthen our relationship with our intuition. The shaking practice's seemingly random nature helps us become more in tune with what our bodies intuitively need to release. Practicing self-observation without judgment helps us to see more authentically what is in front of us. The more old patterns, beliefs, and stories we shed, the more space we have to hear our inner voices. You'd be surprised how clear and decisive intuition is when it has room to speak. Journaling is a wonderful tool for cultivating our relationship with intuition.

Become more aware of the surprises along your writing journey. The idea you didn't think you could possibly write about. The character who jumped out of the cake wearing a jester's hat. The poem about a tree you've never actually seen in "real" life, but have dreamed over and over again.

Your intuition lends you unique insight into the world and into your writing. Let it be your guide and your companion. When it walks hand in hand with you, it will support you. When it feels ignored, it will sabotage you. Intuition is a vital part of what makes us human. Don't disconnect from your intuition in favor of plans and outlines. Likewise, don't dismiss the outline. Use all the tools available to you. Resist the tendency to fracture and rank things according to perceived value. A hammer is not more or less valuable than a wrench. Use everything you've been blessed with on this journey.

## CHAPTER 27

# Resistance Is Futile

Control is never achieved when sought after directly.
It is the surprising outcome of letting go.

—James Arthur Ray

Writing is hard work. I can't present an authentic book on writing that tells you it is easy. Lots of people start on the path and then turn back. Lots of people buy a journal, open it up, and then close it, lest they be blinded by the sheer brightness of the blank page. The Writing Warrior stands steady. Your practice has shown you how to discern illusion from authenticity. Your practice has taught you to trust yourself and to notice what is arising without judgment. You know this too shall pass. All you must do is show up. Try and ignore the stories and poems that are bubbling up inside you. Just try. You can shut them away with distractions. Diversions. But sooner or later, the stories in you waiting for expression will make themselves undeniably known. The path is easier if you don't fight what you've been given. But know this, if you choose to walk the Writing Warrior path, you will meet resistance.

Resistance manifests as tension in the body. This is easy to see in yourself. Try to push against the outside wall of your house. You're pushing with force (resistance) against a structure that is pushing back with exactly the same amount of resistance. Your house may not actually be moving with fingers and arms, but the energy you're sending into the house is being absorbed and pushed back out at you. You'll push all day and the next day and the next until you collapse. Neither of you is going anywhere. You can observe your muscles tightening, your belly constricting, your shoulders rising up to your ears as you push and push in a futile attempt to move your house with your hands. You can see this right away in your body. Resistance and tension in the body are contractions. They take up space. As you lose spaciousness within your body, you lose the ability to flow with what is occurring.

Let's look at resistance in a philosophical way. Yes, on the surface you're resisting the wall of your house. You want it to be in a different place than it is, so you are fighting it. But what's underneath resistance is an unwillingness to accept the way things are. If you first tried accepting the way the wall currently is, you'd have one less boundary in the way of finding a different place for the wall. Acceptance—a surrendering to what is—will make space for you to constructively problem solve. Rather than use all your energy to fight pure strength against pure strength, accept the current reality of the situation and use that energy you would have used to fight to examine other ways of changing the scene.

Surrendering creates space. Think about your body again. When you relax into bed after a long day, you're surrendering everything to the mattress. You're letting go of all the holding and all the tension in your muscles, joints, and bones. You surrender that energy to the earth, and the earth returns it to you by holding you in her cradle. You are then able to take the energy the earth is giving you and use it, rather than expend it.

So what does this have to do with writing? Well, let's look at the gazillion ways each of us likely has for resisting what is surfacing in our work. Go ahead and make a list now. OK. What did you discover?

Resistance is going to feel slightly different in each person, but for me, I feel like I'm digging my heels into the earth. I feel a contraction of the breath and a tightening of the jaw. I notice my mind beginning to attach to anything other than the next sentence in the paragraph. *Wow. I should take a look at cleaning those blinds. Wonder where that book is I was planning to use for my class next semester? Do I need to order some more (fill in the blank) from (fill in the blank)? Has it been only three minutes since I last checked my e-mail? Maybe I just won the National Book Award. Wait, no I wasn't nominated for the National Book Award. I'll never be nominated for the National Book Award. Why doesn't anyone appreciate my writing? I'm a terrible writer, that's why.* And so the threads spin away.

Resistance occurs for many reasons, and it's worth exploring on your own what those reasons might be so you can better recognize them. But underneath that initial resistance lies a fear. The fear takes control of the flow and creates a resistance, which blocks energy, contracts muscles, and then stops work.

Instead, try this. Say you're about to write a scene in which your protagonist must get from the mailbox to her office. It's mostly a set-up scene, but it's important because along the way she's going to encounter someone for the first time who will be significant later. You don't really want to write it because the person she's going to encounter is a loosely disguised version of your mother and you just got off the phone with her a few hours ago and you swear you're about two seconds away from a nervous breakdown. Or the scene bores you, but you know it has to be written or people will be confused. Or you don't yet know enough about your protagonist; for example, why does she need to get from her mailbox to the office so quickly on that particular day? What is so urgent? What is different?

Return to the idea of surrender. What is the next right thing to write? What is the next step in this character's arc? The actual next step, not the step that you believe will get her to the next place you feel she needs to be. By writing small, by staying in intimate contact with the words on the page, you'll maintain a place of flow. By resisting the next word, you'll create contraction.

Don't expend needless energy in resistance to what is surfacing. Accept what you are being given to write and be grateful for it. Many people will never have the luxury or the opportunity or even the ability to write. Don't fight what you're being given. Use its energy to further your own work. In this way, rather than feeling depleted by your writing, you will be filled up by it.

# THE WRITING WARRIOR PRACTICE

I know you've heard it a thousand times before.
But it's true—hard work pays off. If you want to be
good, you have to practice, practice, practice. If you
don't love something, then don't do it.

—Ray Bradbury

Part 4, Committing to Your Authentic Path, has provided you with tools for identifying and releasing illusions and obstacles on the writer's path. We discussed softening our bodies and our inner eyes so we can view ourselves honestly without judgment. We examined the shifting nature of memory and how it affects the way we currently move in the world. Learning to trust your intuition and soften your eyes will also help you revise your work more authentically and completely. Surrendering to the work that is in front of you will release tension in your body and in your writing. Pay attention to your direct experience. Honor it completely.

We tend to experience the deepest resistance when we are about to make the biggest breakthroughs. As a Writing Warrior, stand steady. Use your tools—breathing, shaking, and writing—to dissolve blocks on your path. If you hit something during your writing process that scares you, step back, breathe deeply, and shake it loose. Return to the page cleaner and freer. Take ownership of your journey. Refuse to be a victim to writer's block. Refuse to be chained by your own hands.

## INTERNAL CONVERSATIONS

*You can use the following internal conversation exercises for personal work. The deeper your relationship with yourself, the deeper your writing becomes. Feel free to use poetry or prose to respond.*

Let's practice self-observation without judgment. Sit comfortably in front of a mirror. Allow your gaze to soften as you look at yourself. Notice your thoughts. Are you judging your face? Your wrinkles? Your age spots? Notice, but don't attach. Sit for at least ten minutes gazing at yourself. When you're finished, free write for at least ten minutes. Then find a photograph of yourself from a different time. Sit with this photograph for a minimum of ten minutes. Let your gaze soften as you look at it. Relax your jaw. Soften your shoulders as you relate once again to this person you used to be. When you feel complete, free write for a minimum of ten minutes.

Where do you get in your own way with your self-judgment? What do you think you should have/would have/could have done already? How do those beliefs feel? Write a scene in which you let at least one of them go.

Free write beginning with the phrase: *Absolute vulnerability means . . .* Find an image that conveys absolute vulnerability to you. How do you relate to that image?

In your journal, explore the phrase "soften your shell." Describe your shell. Be specific. What is its texture? Width?

Strength? Location on your body? When did the shell begin forming? How does it benefit you? What is it keeping you from doing? (Remember: self-observation without judgment.)

In your journal, begin with this phrase: "Perhaps you never did _____, but I remember it just the same." What do you remember? What do you know? Are you sure?

Accept that revision is a natural part of the writing process, not something you have to do because you didn't write it right the first time. What is your initial reaction to the idea of revision? Love it? Hate it? Feel too overwhelmed by it?

Set aside thirty minutes to write. You can write anything—a journal entry, a novel, a poem, a blog—it doesn't matter. Your only objective is to write. Keep a separate piece of paper where you can make tick marks. Set your timer for thirty minutes and then go. Notice each time that you've gotten off track (and this takes many forms—switching from your Word doc to a website to shop, checking e-mail, thinking about what you're going to do for dinner, wondering if the sexy guy from the corner store is going to call you back, thinking about the last time you saw your mother); notice anything that pulls you out of the train of word to word that you're writing. Each time you notice that you've been distracted (and you will likely at first *not* notice when it begins; you'll notice it after a few seconds or minutes when you realize you've been holding your hands above the keyboard while your mind has been someplace else), make a tick mark on your piece of paper. When the timer dings at thirty minutes, notice how many tick marks you have. Just notice. Don't judge. The more you practice this, the more tick marks you're going to have, not because you're sliding backward toward sleep, but because you're waking up and observing more quickly when a distraction first occurs. This is requiring your mind to step up its game to keep pace with you.

Over time, the number of tick marks will decrease, but they won't go away all together. Remember: You're not killing the mind. You're integrating the mind.

What were your formative experiences with writing? Diaries? Poetry? A school assignment? Can you identify the moment in your life when writing took on a powerful role? Write that scene.

WRITE NOW

*The following exercises can be applied to works in progress or used as prewriting. Feel free to use poetry or prose to respond.*

Identify a piece of your writing that needs attention and compassion. Read through it (no judgment, just detached scrutiny). Make a plan for what needs to happen to take the work to the next level. Make sure the plan is specific. For example: More research on seventeenth-century modes of transportation. Deepen John's motivation. Cut the scenes with Karen and her cat.

Pick a character you're having trouble with. Describe the shell your character is carrying. When did it begin forming? What benefit is it providing? What is it preventing your character from doing?

Write a scene in which your character ignores the logical or rational course of action and follows his or her intuition. What happens? Be specific.

Fully embody one of the characters you're struggling with. Inhale and exhale with your character. Where is there tightness in your character's body? Write it down. Where are there aches and pains? Write them down. Where does your character feel free and flexible? Write it down. Write a scene focusing only on this character's movement. Your character might be walking through a park or a mall or to the bus stop. Be in your character's body. Nothing else has to happen except physical movement. How does it feel to be moving as someone else?

Examine your characters' relationships with intimacy. Dogen says, "Enlightenment is just intimacy with all things." How does this idea strike your characters? Who and what is your character intimate with?

Embody one of your characters as he or she gazes at himself or herself in the mirror. Describe not just what you see on the surface, but what you see underneath the surface. Look for the story underneath the story.

Your character has a prized object in his or her room. What is it? Describe it. Then view it with soft eyes. How did it come to be in your character's possession? Where was it before then? What does it want to tell your character?

## PART FIVE

# Deepening Your Writer's Roots

## CHAPTER 28

# Alchemy

It is the function of art to renew our perception.
What we are familiar with we cease to see. The
writer shakes up the familiar scene, and, as if by
magic, we see a new meaning in it.

—Anaïs Nin

Ask any writer to explain what it is about his or her
writing that makes it unique. You'll get some stum-
bling, some searching. *Perhaps my voice? My ideas?*
But a writer knows that those things are only part of the
answer. The rest of the answer is a mystery. It's that mystery
that keeps us coming back to the page. What's going to happen today? Who am I going to meet? What are they going to
say? What am I going to learn? How is my life going to be
changed by this story? Who is going to show up?

These questions pull us from the bed to the computer
at five in the morning so we can write before going to the
office. They tug us away from a staff meeting to jot down
notes on a poem. They keep us in that childlike place of curi-
osity and compassion. Who? What? When? Where? Why?
We don't know, and so we write to find out.

The magic part of the writing process is different for each
writer. All the parts of an art form cannot be quantified in a

book or a class. For the most part, we can collectively agree on mechanics. On several ways to build tension. On paying attention to adverb usage. But we can't collectively agree on where the voices and stories come from. And that, to me, is what makes the whole journey worthwhile.

I love to talk with other writers about their creative process. Do you hear voices? What do you see? What questions are haunting you? What emotions bang against your ribs at night? What characters have you lived with your whole life? Being able to have conversations with people who don't run out of the room or call 911 when you ask these questions is an important part of a writer's life. It's nice to know we're not crazy (or at least not dangerously so!). And it's vital to honor this not-knowing part of writing.

Voices and places are often the catalysts for my stories. I'll hear a line or two, or even a sound of someone's voice. Perhaps I'll see a house and a landscape. It's no coincidence that my two strongest writing gifts are dialogue and setting. Pay attention to your own inner wisdom, pay attention to how writing shows up for you. Do you hear a voice or see a scene? Does an idea that needs to be explored present itself? When you're aware of your inner voice, you'll hear it more often. When you're aware of how your stories come to you, you'll recognize them more quickly.

Think of alchemy as the art of transformation. Early alchemists tried to change common metals into gold and silver using heat. As writers, we take the common experiences of daily life, bring them into our beings, and transform them into art. Each of us notices and observes the world differently. As our awareness of our observations deepens, our art deepens. As you read this section on the mystery of writing, ask yourself: What is your writer's alchemy? What is carried on your breath? The answers to those questions will point you in the direction your writing wants to take you. Be still and let it guide you.

CHAPTER 29

# Hark! Who Goes There?

The more enlightened our houses are, the more
their walls ooze ghosts.

—Italo Calvino

I n the winter of 2007, I had the privilege of hearing Shantala, a husband and wife duo, perform at my yoga studio.
The room was filled, so filled in fact that we steam etched
the windows (an odd occurrence for Arizona!). We "aum'd"
them in and then sang with them for ninety minutes. Benji,
who performs backup vocals and percussion, opened with a
dedication of the whole year's performances to his mother,
who had died on Christmas day. "To say it is the hardest
thing I have ever gone through is an understatement," the
fifty-year-old man said. "Her spirit will be dancing with us
tonight in her flannel shirt and Goodwill hat."

We laughed in that way of laughing that hides the sadness. I watched the man next to me brush his hand over
his eyes. The woman on the folding chair in front of me
kept her eyes closed while tears eked out the edges. I imagined Benji's mother's spirit in a flannel shirt dancing with
my father in a golf shirt while we all, those of us embodied
now, re-remembered how fragile our flesh was. Benji talked

of unlikely teachers. He talked of the battles his mother had fought against the government for denying the increased risk of cancer for people living under exposed power lines. He told of her coming to his concerts at eighty years old with her forty (yes, forty) year old boyfriend, tapping her feet and dancing. The greatest way to honor her spirit, he said, was to use his gifts.

Then, they sang.

Helen, one of the protagonists in my current novel *Unbearable Compassion*, circled above them, called, apparently, at the news of the death of Benji's mother. "My mother died when I was eight," Helen whispered to me. "That's why I had to leave Georgia. That's why I couldn't take care of Claire. That's why I killed Ellie."

"You didn't kill Ellie," I whispered back. "You just didn't know how to take care of her."

"My mother lay in her bed dead for three days before anyone came to find her," she said. "I curled up with her." She took a swig of her whiskey. "I curled up with her." She took out her bridge and snarled at me, gums deep red. "Damn you."

I watched her, toothless, drunk, and old, but still eight years old. I watched her watch Benji's mother hover over her son, fingers of light touching his skin. I watched her melt.

"Stop poking at me," Helen said.

I kept chanting, kept listening. I took off my fleece vest. I took off my socks and held my feet.

"There's no Ellie out there, dancing," whispered Helen.

I shook my head. No Ellie. She'd been dead almost forty years. Helen hadn't wanted her.

It's a thread of mothers, I thought. *Unbearable Compassion* is a thread of mothers. How about that.

I have learned to follow visions, obsessions, and quirky bits of intuition. I am one day obsessed with old Southern juke joints. I feel myself in them, swaying, dancing, sweating.

I see the singer, a thin black woman with long fingers in a dress so red it shouts. I feel the music walk up my spine, though the kind of blues she's singing about I've never known. I see the knife carvings in the tables, the red clay mud on the floor. I've never been in a juke joint, but one morning I wake up and am surrounded by characters I don't recognize, but a sound my soul remembers. What is this?

One day, it is tulips. I order books about them. I take pictures of them. I study their bulbs. Their many colors. I read up on Holland. Why? One day, in my mind, I watch a little boy being buried on his family's farmland in south Georgia. The father makes the coffin himself the night before. He worked alone in the woodshed while his wife baked and baked and baked. His other son has taken off again for the lake. His other son who has not drowned has returned to the place where the drowning occurred. The place where he did not pay attention. He has removed his shoes before stepping first one foot then the other into the dark lake, but he is not brave enough to follow his brother. Or he is not guilty enough. He'll spend his lifetime wondering which.

Images appear and disappear. Voices whisper just on the other side of the wall. The story unfolds in front of you too quickly to capture, so you wait until it shows itself again. I don't know where they come from. I only know they do come, and the longer you stay put and wait, the more frequently you'll see them. Don't analyze the gifts that appear. Instead, hold them in your hand as if they were a pair of monarch butterflies. Watch the delicate wings. Notice the antennae, the feather-like texture of the colors. Trust yourself to write the next right word without thinking about it. Trust yourself to write the next right scene. It will emerge from the scene in front of it. Listen to its pulse and follow its lead. Practice this active listening and notice what changes in your writing.

I taught writing groups at a local Girl Scout camp for several summers. We were doing a listening activity one day when a girl with thick glasses shouted, "I have voices in my head!" Rather than make fun of her, the other young writers at the table merely nodded.

"We all do," said another girl.

"Yeah," said the girl with the thick glasses. "But I didn't know they were so *loud*."

## CHAPTER 30

# I-10 between Phoenix and Tucson

> Most people think that shadows follow, precede
> or surround beings or objects. The truth is that
> they also surround words, ideas, desires, deeds,
> impulses and memories.
>
> —Elie Wiesel

I travel east on I-10 past mile after mile of broken glass, tire skins, rusted axles, and brown dirt and wonder how anyone could ever say there is nothing on this road. I went to college in Tucson, and every time I travel this stretch, I feel out of balance. Some years, leaving Phoenix and driving to Tucson was going home. Other years, the opposite.

Cars filled with eighteen-year-olds off to college jam the road. Possibilities stretch in dotted lines in front of them. Retirees from Minnesota driving motor homes bigger than my house inch over the lane markings. The road behind them releases regrets.

Altars speckle I-10. Crosses edged with carnations, candles, letters, and balloons are monuments signifying that at that spot someone's life changed forever. My own crosses are not marked with wooden sticks and hand-lettered signs, but I see them three-dimensionally every time I make this trip on this road where I grew up, grew apart, grew together.

On the way to Tucson, I gather the ghosts. Sacatan Rest Area, with its brown round restrooms and vending machines and warnings about dangerous insects and snakes is where I pick up the first one. She's nineteen and bitter. Fire cracks in her eyes. She just buried her father. Just left her family. She climbs into the backseat, smacks her spearmint gum, pops a few M&M's in her mouth, and stares at the back of my head. We pull out of the rest area and are reminded to Buckle Up: It's the Law. The ghost looks out the window, yawns, and refuses to put on her seatbelt. It's seventy-eight miles to Tucson. We'll have a long time to chat.

I almost died at mile marker 199, where the second ghost jumps in, east of Casa Grande. Looks like an ordinary roadside, with the stray Adidas tennis shoe upside down in the dust and the coyote bones bleached almost clear, patches of the animal's tan fur pressed into the dirt. Along the highway's edge, the road dissolves to gravel. I was tired. Driving in the dark. Going back to college. Fell asleep. A semitruck behind me flashed its brights and honked its horn, and my head jerked up and awake, my car swerving inches from the mile marker sign and a wooden fence post. I spun in the gravel on the shoulder and stopped, heart pumping, hair electric, palms sticky. I rolled the window down and smelled the asphalt and musky heat. Even with cars passing in both directions, I knew the land around me was deep enough to walk into and vanish, wrapped in a cloak of indigo night.

The second ghost has only one tennis shoe and hair so short she's almost bald. Her mouth is stitched closed. She kicks the same things over and over with her bare foot and cries when her toes bruise. Time to wake up. Remain present. Accountable.

The third ghost lives at Toltec outside the Carl's Jr. She waits, drinking an up-sized Diet Coke at the yellow plastic table, for me to pick her up. She's got a ferret, a brand-new college degree, and bright red hair. Her ring finger is bare, but the suntan line still glows from the diamond she wore for two years. She comes to sit in the passenger seat, looking warily at the ghosts in the back. She hates them. She turns the radio to the pop station. I smile and ease the dial over a few notches. She doesn't realize that the modern music she's looking for has somehow become classic rock. She moves back into the backseat, and I pull out of the parking lot and wait for a caravan of Wal-Mart trucks to enter the on-ramp in front of me. They spit black smoke into the air. The red-headed ghost coughs and drums the riff to a Foreigner song on her legs.

The fourth ghost hitchhikes on the hill just outside of Marana, where the high school stretches into the middle school and farther down to the playground of the grade school. Cops wait here to catch speeders. This ghost smiles and waves. She's jumping into a new life, a new future, a new home. She's hopeful, hoping. She squeezes into the backseat and the whole energy of the car shifts. I like this one. I remember her. She still wanted to play.

The ghosts ride with me into Tucson and through it. Past U of A, where I hardly recognize the campus anymore, and the signs above the construction zones tell me my mother's tuition dollars are still hard at work. Past my old two-room apartment with the lima bean-green door where I learned more in a year about what I would not tolerate than at any other time in my life. Past Greasy Tony's where we'd eat Philly cheesesteak sandwiches and french fries as if our metabolism would never change, and we would always have hours in the afternoons to talk about Woolf and Faulkner.

Back to Phoenix and the car is heavy, carrying all the

excess. I feel it in my shoulders. I hear it in the whine of the four-cylinder engine shifting gears as we go from zero to seventy-five as quickly as my little Sentra can.

Let them go. Let them go.

Shells of buildings litter I-10. The Picacho Motel is nothing but a monolithic sign in front of dust. The Precision Machine Shop just east of State Route 87 stands empty, the glass in the window coated with green dust. Train tracks run both east and west along I-10's westbound side. Cargo trains pull double-decker loads of boxcars painted yellow and gray past crossings where the red lights flash to warn no cars of its approach.

I wonder who stops and buys genuine Indian jewelry at the Dairy Queen off of exit 219. Who buys the "real" Mexican blankets and the Black Hills gold? Who stops along the edge of a speeding highway to breathe in the dust of trucks and travelers and eat a banana split and trade journey stories with the man behind the counter? Seekers. People searching for their stories. Thinking perhaps a bit of history in the form of petrified rock bookends or leather moccasins might answer some of the deeper questions of their hearts.

In the backseat, all four ghosts sleep in each other's arms. The car is quiet, the whining of the engine vanished. I watch them in the rearview mirror, breathing together. I pull into a rest area and stop the car.

"Hey," I whisper. "Move on now."

They wake up, a collective quad of self-reflections, and slip through the door into the desert. The car smells of vanilla. I move forward, zero to seventy-five in record time. I breathe.

People say there's nothing on this stretch of road. Nothing much, maybe. Just everything I've ever been, and the possibilities of everything I am to be. The mountains in front of me are rimmed in magenta and burnt umber. The sky is gray to the south, baby blue to the north. Dust winds a serpentine path upward. Ahead of me, the sun.

What ghosts line the highways of your life? Which ghosts can you pick up? Which ones can you discard? Which ones have you ignored and which ones have you canonized? Pay attention with absolute vulnerability and compassion. Listen with your heart, and then pick up your pen.

We are the sum of all we have been. Understanding and integrating the people we have been throughout a lifetime is an important part of the writer's alchemy. The more whole we are, the deeper we can go in our writing. We've all been through stages and phases in our lives. We've likely gone through many shifts—in what we want for our lives, who we want to attract, and who we strive to be. Just like each draft of a story is perfect unto itself, so is each incarnation we've had along life's path. All you have been is perfect. Gather your fractured selves together, breathe them in, and transform them. Use their fuel to create something new.

## CHAPTER 31

# Writing Is Not Like Making a Peanut Butter and Jelly Sandwich

> Every sentence has a truth waiting at the end of it, and the writer learns how to know it when he finally gets there.
>
> —Don DeLillo

Every single time you sit down to write—a story, a poem, an essay, a novel—it will be a brand-new experience. No formula works. The mystery that solved your previous story doesn't speak the same language as your current story. The key that unlocked the sonnet of yesterday won't work today. Accept that. Don't resist it. Writing never works the same way twice. You can view this as exciting or frustrating. Or, you can accept it for what it is. The writing process.

Writing is not like making a peanut butter and jelly sandwich. All the ingredients are not waiting for you in the cupboard. You—armed with skill and the memory of successful past peanut butter and jelly-making performances, and knowing that, barring the absence of a key ingredient, like say, peanut butter or bread, you'll be able to deliver a delicious sandwich, a sandwich just as delicious as the one you made yesterday, or last week, or when you were twelve—feel success as a peanut-butter-and-jelly-sandwich-maker extraordinaire. Writing is not in any way like this. The longer you believe that it is, the longer you will struggle needlessly.

Writing is not in any way like assembling a car engine. Or baking a cake. Or aligning your body for the perfect golf swing. The longer you believe that it is, the longer you will struggle needlessly.

I can't tell you how much I *want* writing to be like these things. Even after all these years of writing and teaching, I still can get suckered into believing that someone has "an answer," and if only I'd do this or that or the other thing, I'd finally get it. And every time I get suckered, I vow never to be suckered again. There's always a promise of something that will solve The Writer's Problem.

This book is not making that promise. That's an inauthentic promise. No matter how much discipline we have, no matter how many tools we've gathered, we still need to figure out our practice anew each time we sit down to write. Understanding this will help you avoid frustration and deepen your roots as a writer.

Writing can never be like making a peanut butter and jelly sandwich because your ingredients aren't sitting on a shelf waiting for you to take them down. If writing were truly like making a peanut butter and jelly sandwich, first you'd have to plant the seeds to grow the wheat to make the bread. Grow the peanuts to make the butter. Pick the fruit to make the jelly. Decide if you want white, wheat, sourdough, rye, or pumpernickel. Decide if you want chunky or smooth. Apple or grape or strawberry. Then realize you can't always get what you want. Sometimes the harvest doesn't come in and there's not enough wheat for the bread. Sometimes worms get the apples and there's no jelly. You can't know these things though, until you're all set and ready to make your sandwich—nay, until you're in mid-sandwich-making-mode—and then you learn there are no strawberries. Or no peanuts. Or the bread went stale. Or there are only the ends and you hate the ends.

Sometimes you don't know these things until you get quite far into the process. And then you're frustrated and decide peanut butter sandwiches are stupid anyway. There are far too many peanut butter and jelly sandwiches in the world. Far too many people. Too many peanuts. Too many grapes to make the jelly with, and far, far too much bread. Storehouses of grain for loaves upon loaves of bread. Go be a farmer. A doctor. A preacher. A snake oil salesman. Anything, anything, but a writer. A maker of original peanut butter and jelly sandwiches. Really, you say to yourself, what can you possibly have to offer that hasn't already been done and done better than you could ever imagine?

Stop. Breathe. Pick up your pen. Raise your fingers above your keyboard. Just start already. The world is hungry for what only you can create.

## CHAPTER 32

# Sand Paintings

The writer's duty is to keep on writing.

—William Styron

Tibetan Buddhist monks spend weeks and months creating intricate sand paintings only to brush them away at the end of their labor. The process of creation and destruction is a sacred meditation in nonattachment. Three days ago, I was working on two scenes from my novel. The writing was working. It wasn't great, but it was good draft work. Two days ago, I was working on the scene that followed those scenes when my computer froze, forcing me to do a reset, which caused (though it wasn't supposed to cause this) a loss of all my data. I had a portion of the book saved on a different computer, and though this computer freeze didn't make me jump for joy, it was only about ten hours of work and I looked at it (mostly) as an opportunity to revise and make the scenes better. I always advise my students to take their early drafts and put them in a drawer and not look at them as they move into the revision process. I believe revision is best done on a fresh piece of paper. So I figured this was a chance for me to practice that in a little more of a boot camp fashion than I was accustomed to. I went home, wrote a quick outline of everything I'd written, taking special care to write down the surprise details that came up during the process of writing. Not that big a deal.

Today, I had four hours to work this afternoon. I was able to rewrite the scenes that had been lost as well as move forward two more scenes. And yes, you guessed it, the screen froze again. What an opportunity to practice my yoga, I thought, as I wanted to throw this machine across the room. What a teacher this computer is turning out to be. What is this actually about? I've never lost data in my life, and now it's happened twice in one week. By the time I rewrite the scenes tomorrow (on a different computer), they'll be pretty darn fine scenes.

My first thought, after "oh shit," was of the Tibetan monks and their beautiful sand paintings. I remembered reading an interview in which they were asked why they spent all that time making the mandalas only to destroy them. They replied, as monks are wont to do, that the making of the mandala was what mattered, not what happened to it after it was finished.

"But how can you work so hard to make it so beautiful knowing it will be gone in a few weeks?"

"The work is the practice. That is all there is. Everything else is an illusion. Today we make a painting. Tomorrow it is gone. This is the way of everything."

So tomorrow, when I rewrite those scenes again, and back them up on two thumb drives and e-mail them to myself at work, I'll approach them with that frame of mind. I can never rewrite them like I wrote them the first time. Some images are gone. The ones that matter will come back. New ones will appear. This is the way of everything. When the sand paintings blush with color, and when they vanish on the winds of breath.

## CHAPTER 33

# The Beginning Is
# Not the Beginning

One should be able to return to the first sentence of a novel and find the resonances of the entire work.

—Gloria Naylor

Someday maybe you'll write my story, hey, sugar?" Dad was lying on his left side on his bed, thumbing through a scrapbook I had made for him that contained all his golf tournament clippings, his school musical programs, his wedding announcement in the Wilmington paper, even a piece of desk stationery from his tenure at Blue Cross Blue Shield. If he held any nostalgia about any of the clippings, he didn't let on then. He paused in front of the photo of him at age eight, in white baggy underwear, trying to walk again after the polio left (or so we thought). He was the face of polio for Wilmington, the boy in the photo spread intended to help raise money for the March of Dimes' fight for the cure. His gaze reflected both bewilderment and a steady focus.

He closed the scrapbook. "A lot has happened since then."

"I'll write your story," I said, not knowing what that promise would mean for me. I was seventeen then.

I didn't see that scrapbook again until years after his death and my mother's remarriage. When I held it in my hands the next time, I was once again seventeen, still trying to freeze the moments of his life. My desire to chronicle in impressive detail the events that made up his life caught me again like the firefly in the Mason jar. In trying so hard to keep everything from changing, the light died, and I was left with black-and-white newsprint photos and articles that captured just the skeleton of his life, and were as dead as he was. This wasn't his story; it was just a catalog of the things he did. These listings didn't tell me anything about him, except that he had polio in 1948, was an exceptional golfer, went to Wake Forest and Chapel Hill, married Elinor Ranta, a Lutheran from Brooklyn, in 1965, and sold insurance for Blue Cross Blue Shield. The scrapbook, like his life in some ways, ended after his heart attack in 1976. How must it have made him feel to receive a scrapbook of his life that ended while he was under thirty? To me, as a teenager making the book for him, it seemed like he'd already had a long and full life. Now, as I edge over forty, I taste the bitter saliva of its brevity.

When Dad died, I put a piece of thin typing paper into my IBM Selectric and began:

My father was the greatest man I've ever known.

I wrote pages in this vein, trying to get down everything I possibly could before I forgot. Trying to freeze-frame my nineteen years with him. The pages, filled with hero worship and unresolved grief, may represent an authentic capturing of the moment, but they don't represent good writing. I was trying too hard, wanting too much to be the historian, attaching hard edges of distance to the scenes so that no one could know my father from those words. I wanted to preserve him only for me. In order for me to write in such a way that the reader could get to know him, I would have to let him go.

I wrote about fifty pages in 1987 and then put them in my desk drawer. I couldn't do it. I felt terrible giving up on writing about my dad, but I didn't know what to do about it, and, frankly, I was already tired of the blandness of grief. That's something they don't tell you; grief is stark as a prairie. Occasionally a fire rushes through, or a flood, but most days, it's the same—beating sun, shrinking cold, and endless, endless sky.

His story was never going to work as long as I continued to circle around an ideal and an idea of what had happened. It was never going to work as long as I refused to let Dad move. I've now lived longer without him than with him. I don't know that I can claim to have known him at all. My sister and I consistently have different ideas of what he would or wouldn't have done in a given situation. This makes sense; we each knew a different man, and we're both different people, so we resonated with different parts of his personality. I had to realize I couldn't write *his* story, I could only write his story in relationship to mine. And I couldn't do that until I had the key components to any story: action, motion, movement. I could stay in the cocoon of frozen animation forever if I wanted to, but there would be no book, no story, no life—for me or for him.

Every novel or story I have ever written begins this way. First, the intellect. The fear of loss if I don't get down the "idea," the main points, the theme—the desperation of a theme. *I have to write my father's story because if I don't, no one will remember him, and if no one remembers him, then no one will remember me.* Sticky. Laden with expectations and intentions. Burdened with an impossible mission statement. Beware of writing themes. They cling to your throat like fish netting.

Don't try to write *about* anything. Instead, write from direct experience of the story as it unfolds in front of you. Release any desire for a specific result. Let the story speak. Shake yourself loose, leaving only the writing pulsing, present, and alive.

After almost twenty years of writing seriously, I now move much more quickly through this place of mandates. I catch myself after a few weeks; *oh yeah, Laraine, get out of your head. Oh right, who do you really think you are? Just shut up and listen already.*

CHAPTER 34

# Sacred Communication

An artist is a creature driven by demons. He doesn't know why they choose him and he's usually too busy to wonder why.

—William Faulkner

I have been thinking about how trapped our characters must feel within the pages of a book—bound, as it were, by the spine, crushed by the cover. Dead until a reader cracks the spine and breaks the chains, allowing the reader's imagination to merge with the characters' lives. Maybe there's a connection. Maybe there isn't. Inevitably, the book must close, the characters sprawled and pressed flat like dried flowers.

As writers, we give the gift of impermanence to our readers. We allow them to step into a world for a few hours or a few weeks, then step out, changed. We allow them to practice loving fully the people who dance in the sentences. We give them the practice of letting the characters go. Each novel a reader enters teaches detachment and absolute vulnerability if the reader is brave enough to face herself in the pages.

Each novel we write gives us these same gifts. We open our lungs, livers, and spleens and listen to who speaks to us. We notice the ache in our femur and stop to talk to whoever is stuck there. We loosen our jaws to speak what we have been afraid to speak, or unwilling to speak. We relax our wrists, position our fingers over the keyboard, breathe in, and then exhale out with the sound of stories. We listen more deeply when we begin to get in our way. We find ourselves writing things we didn't know we felt, things we didn't know were possible. These characters, once awakened, swirl in our dreams. They influence our outward behavior, our interests, and our hobbies. They pull us into unexpected shops or towns. We follow because it is what we writers do.

And then these relationships, longer perhaps than many of our "human" ones, dissolve. They have spoken what they have to say. We have listened to what we can hear. We have built the bridge of letters between them and the rest of the world. What happens to them is no longer a part of our lives. We detach from them, or perhaps more accurately, they detach from us and we wander a bit lost for a while, missing them, wondering why we are missing them, wondering why they didn't want to stay longer. We haunt our own hallways searching for them.

But then, if we have practiced detachment, a tickle appears at the base of our spines. A sudden obsession with peaches, or the Industrial Revolution, or ant colonies. We follow intuition until a sound cracks through and our fingers sing once again.

Among the countless reasons that writing matters, this is the most important to me. Writing teaches impermanence. It shows us how to move with ease from one chapter of our lives to another. It provides practice for our ultimate transition. It embodies, on the recycled flesh of trees, what is most beautiful, most holy, and most possible within us. Open the book's covers wide and let my characters move.

Open the book's covers wide and let your hearts and minds expand. Open the book's covers wide and step back with awe and gratitude for the part of all of us that creates, that risks, and that ultimately, bids us a most fond and joyous farewell.

## CHAPTER 35

# Characters as Teachers

I don't want to say I hear voices; well, actually, I
do hear voices, but I don't think it's supernatu-
ral. I think it's just that when characters are given
enough texture and backbone, then lo and behold,
they stand on their own.

—Anne Tyler

The moon waxes outside my bedroom window. Thumb
Butte is silhouetted in grays. Tonight there are bats
and coyotes and tiny biting bugs. I smell javelina,
though I haven't seen one rutting around the scrub brush
in quite some time. I'm awake at my usual time—3:45 AM.
I watch and listen. Sometimes I wake up and just use the
bathroom. Sometimes I wake up and pull whichever cat is
closer under the covers with me. I can usually get away with
that for a few minutes before she gets sick of me and jumps
away. But other times, I wake up because something has
shown up—a solution to a scene in a novel, a new book idea,
a sadness that seems real only at 3:45 AM.

"Hey," says Lillian, one of my characters. "Don't let us
keep you awake." She presses her hand to my forehead,

sinking me back onto the pillow. I burrow deeper under the down.

"Wake up!" It's Hannah, another character. "I've still got more to say to you."

"Shut up." This one's Zöe, the one who's way too much like me. "You had your turn. It's my turn now."

"Ain't none of y'all's turn," says Frank, from my newest novel. "It's my time now. I'm still stuck in Chinatown."

I could be asleep, but I'm not. The bed is heavy with all of them here. More are here than choose to speak. There are always more of them than are speaking. Always more.

Two black swans slide across a pond I can't identify. I think of Freedom Park in North Carolina where we used to go when I was growing up to feed the ducks and crows. I wonder what those black swans are about. Janis Joplin cracks her heart open in Golden Gate Park in 1967 and twenty-year-old Helen feels the blood thumping in her own heart. In her belly, a baby who won't live to hear Janis wailing. Outside the park, Benjamin, another ghost, circles over Frank's head in Chinatown. The ghosts of my characters.

Skeleton Woman dances on the dresser, the moon casting her reflection in the mirror, a sight beautiful enough to make me eternally grateful for this life. She nods at me, her jaw a constant grin.

No character has ever visited me who didn't have something to teach me. No story ever moved through me that didn't help me move. I have learned this through years of observing my writing and my relationship with it. Knowing that every character, every story or poem teaches me something helps me to get out of my own way. It helps me continue to have faith in what I'm working on even when I can't see where it's going. Paying attention and waking up to the lessons of each book and character help me stay more present in my work. It helps me release my desire for a result because I've witnessed over and over that the work knows more than I do. I know that if I make a space for it, writing will take me places I cannot conceive of on my own.

The cats sleep in fluffy cat piles. The black swans slide across the surface of the lake. I close my eyes to dream a story. My characters gather around. "We're here, love."

My bones sing. What a wondrous gift indeed, to be one of the haunted.

CHAPTER 36

# Let's Do the Limbo

When having a smackerel of something with a friend, don't eat so much that you get stuck in the doorway trying to get out.

—Winnie the Pooh

Nothing's more fun than realizing you're smack dab in the middle of the very place and space you talk to your students about all the time. On the one hand, it validates your discussion. On the other hand, it just plain sucks.

I've started four different novels in the last three months, none of which seem to be going anywhere. I do know enough to know that I need to keep following them, but the honest truth is that I am extremely lonely when I'm not living with a bunch of characters. I feel incomplete. I feel like I'm searching for the rest of me.

I received an anonymous postcard this week. I've gotten a few of these over the last year or so. The postmark is Vermont. I don't know anyone in Vermont, so I'm kind of excited to have a secret Vermont admirer. The postcard said: *If your train doesn't pull into the station, go out and find it*. Very appropriate for the past few months. Of course, the next logical question is: Go where? Go west, young (ahem, middle-aged) woman, go west? Go east? Go north, south, inside, outside, upside down, underneath . . . Ah, so many prepositions, so little time. But the gist is: move.

Writing limbo takes many forms. Waiting for the characters to speak. Waiting for that call from an agent or editor. Waiting for the answer to your plot conundrum. But waiting isn't inertia. Inertia will beget inertia, and before you know it, you'll have a whole inertia dynasty lounging around your house. You'll be overwhelmed. All the inertia siblings will be fighting over the remote control. Don't let it get that far. When you find yourself stuck, shake. Move. Walk. Run. Cycle. Don't let the weight of inertia, which is just a spoke on our Writer's Wheel of Suffering, keep you motionless.

You have no control over when your editor will call. You have no control over when that plot solution will show up. There's no tracking number on those things. Break your expectations apart. Change your approach. Rather than ask the question you think you want the answer to (How will Bernard ever get out of the mine shaft in New Mexico?), instead ask Bernard what he's thinking while he's stuck in the mine shaft. Let Bernard show you the way out. Ask Bernard what the next right thing for him to do is. Don't try so hard to make it happen by yourself.

In some versions of Chinese mythology, the afterlife contains a viewing pavilion where hungry ghosts are sent to watch their families. The ghosts can't interact with their loved ones. They can't help them. They can't change the course of events. They can only watch and wait.

There's a viewing pavilion for us as writers, too. We know a book is out there. We can see its edges, maybe even its title or cover. We might hear a voice or two, see a scene. But we can't touch it. It dances just beyond our reach; in fact, the harder we try to grab it, the more elusive it becomes. Our job is to remain on the viewing pavilion until the book encircles us with its arms and we smell the ink on the page. You'll know the difference between the right time to write and the forced time. Remember the words of Leo Tolstoy. "The two most powerful warriors are patience and time."

During this time of waiting, take notes. Observe your thoughts about the book. Observe your desires, your contractions, and your grasping. Observe what needs you have (need to publish, need to please, need to be famous, need to be rich) and blow them away. Observe your expectations and, one by one, cast them into the sea. We must wait. Waiting is not doing nothing. Waiting prepares you. Waiting creates discipline. Waiting allows you to feel what it's like to break the tension and then birth the ocean of a story. If we could give birth every day, every hour all of our lives, then we would forget to notice the miracle, which is not possible without the period of gestation.

Never is nothing happening. Never are you not in perfect harmony with the work you are supposed to write. Understand this and your writing will open. Fight this and your work will contract. Both places will teach you.

Writing is much more about listening and waiting than it is about writing. Some of my novels have come to me first through a voice in the very back of my mind. I'll get a line, or a fragment of a line. Then maybe the same day, maybe the next year, I'll get more context. Some stories come to me through an image of a place. I don't know how and I don't know why. I have simply learned patience. This doesn't mean I'm not writing during the waiting. I am. I'm exploring, gathering. Like a child taking a basket out into the woods to bring back interesting things, a writer goes out with an empty notebook and gathers without knowing why. Oh, look, a book on Japanese tea ceremonies. "Huh?" says your mind. "You don't care about that." No matter. Put it in your basket.

You pick up a funky peacock feather at the local craft store. "Huh?" No matter. Gather. You're suddenly obsessed with corn necklaces. Just notice. Write it down. Keep shopping.

Remember the words of author Judith Claire Mitchell, "Learn to see and then to listen to the ghosts who come to your writing room." Gather those ghosts to you. Embrace whatever form they take. Don't try to fix them, change them, analyze them, or order them around. Just put them in your basket. Give them a place in your notebook. They may soon whisper to you or they may jump out of the basket and return at a different time. Love them fully, whatever they look like. Whatever they say. They are yours, and you are privileged to be able to hear them.

CHAPTER 37

# Seasons of the Work

To be interested in the changing seasons is a happier state of mind than to be hopelessly in love with spring.

—George Santayana

I am pulled away from the computer this afternoon by the smell of rain blowing through my open window. Water! It is late June in the northern Arizona high desert. Time for monsoon season to begin. The temperature has dropped ten degrees this afternoon, and the cats are glued to the window screen, the breeze dancing with their fur. I step outside. There are only a few drops this afternoon, but they're cold, and there's the slow promise of thunder. It's also wildfire season, and a wildfire is burning about sixty miles southeast. So far, it's charred over one hundred acres. I saw the plume of smoke in the sky yesterday as I drove home from Sedona. This morning, the smoke had blown in over Prescott, raining light ash from the sky. I couldn't see Thumb Butte through the haze.

Monsoon season makes us come out of our houses to stand in the rain. We gaze at the sky, which is so frequently just a sheet of turquoise blue, and point to bushels of clouds.

Wind stirs up the dust from the yard. Lightning brings its fire. A monsoon is a celebration of all the elements, and we, who have so long been deprived of water, can't help but sing.

The absence of defined seasons in Phoenix made that area particularly challenging for me to live in. As the city has grown, it gets fewer monsoon storms, the heat from the cement and the sprawl having altered the weather patterns. Phoenix has highs between 80 and 120 degrees all year long. My body couldn't figure out when to rest, when to work, when to play. Prescott, however, is a mile high, with four full seasons, although none of them are extreme. Winter feels like winter. We need scarves and gloves and heat. We need to sleep more and drink warm liquids and soups. Summer is bright and clear, with daylight lasting twelve hours. We need sunscreen and salads and cool water. Living in Prescott has taught me about the seasons of my own body. I couldn't feel them in Phoenix. I watched as the stores brought in wool and fur coats, gloves, hats, and fleece even though the thermometer read 90 degrees in November.

Writing a book has four seasons, too, although they don't always occur chronologically. Sometimes the seeds you plant are not ready yet, and no amount of watering, watching, or cursing will make the plant grow before it's ready. You cannot force a piece of writing. You may choose to put plastic flowers on your kitchen table, but everyone knows they're plastic flowers.

Discipline in your writing practice will help you listen to its seasons. When is it time to plant? When is it time to gather? When is it time to wait? When is it time to harvest? I understand how seductive the push is to get something done "now." I too have witnessed and experienced the pain of forcing a piece of work to arrive before it's ready. That work will not be healthy. It cannot stand on its own. It cannot show you how to shape it into a book. It doesn't have all the nutrients it needs to be what it was becoming before you cut it out of the earth too early.

In my experience with teaching and writing, books seem to begin first with the powerful force of summer, followed too quickly by the stillness of winter. That stillness can kill a novice writer's enthusiasm for the work. It can bring up doubts, hungry ghosts, and other "better ideas," locking you in an endless summer. But if you hunker down and wait, after winter will come spring, and you will see the green buds of the flurry of work you did in summer begin to surface. As the days get longer, your energy will increase, and the book will begin to pull you again, ever and always farther into your own psyche and the mythology of the story.

Observe how this unfolds in your own work. You might use headings such as "Winter" or "Spring" in your writing journal as you explore your process. Never mind that you are writing "Spring" when it is December. Listen to the work. Its calendar is its own.

CHAPTER 38

# Texas

If we are facing in the right direction, all we have to
do is keep on walking.

—Buddhist proverb

Before our family moved west to Arizona, I had never
been anywhere in the country except up and down
the eastern and southern coasts. What I knew of the
West came from the prairies in the Little House books and
from reruns of *Bonanza* and the country and western sing-
ers Dad liked to listen to: Tex Ritter, George Jones, Waylon
and Willie. My seventh-grade friends wrote in my yearbook
to watch out for scorpions and buffalo and gunfights. This
was what we thought the West was, we children of the South.
We thought it was spiny and dusty and dry, with hangings on
the square and men wearing chaps and six-shooters. We had
our share of poisonous, strange animals in the South, but
I knew what they were, and since I wasn't an outdoors girl,
I was generally safe. Scorpions, apparently, lived in people's
shoes. How could I avoid shoes?

We drove west mostly on I-40. I began to understand why
the Mississippi River was such a prominent dividing line for

the country. Everything east of the Mississippi exploded in greens. Everything west of the Mississippi looked, to me, like an Etch-A-Sketch screen, only there was no way to shake the gray away and make a new picture. We stopped for a night in Henryetta, Oklahoma. The motel had a pool, but the pool water was too green. Our motel room had dark blue velvet bedspreads that seemed exotic to me, and the beds had a coin-operated massage feature. The parking lot was filled with trucks. We heard the sounds from the interstate all night. In the morning, after a breakfast of Cheerios in the motel room, we continued west, the sun behind us.

I-40 travels through the Texas panhandle. Though this is the shortest east-west route through Texas, I thought we would never get through it. I had never seen such barren land. And I didn't want us to get through it, because with every mile we continued west, the odds of turning back east grew slimmer. I was afraid of what would be in Arizona, or, more accurately, what wouldn't be in Arizona. And then there was the thing none of us were talking about; we were moving to Arizona so Dad could die. We all knew he wanted to see us have a better start without him than he thought we could have in North Carolina. But we didn't talk about that, and, looking back, I don't know if it would have made a difference.

I felt, and still feel, vulnerable in the West, unprotected, waiting for the claws of a hawk to clamp to the back of my neck and carry me off. The space is too wide, the sky too endless, the trees too short. In the south, trees that witnessed slavery still stand tall and solid. Trees there have arms that reach above me and below me, their roots twisting, turning, joining under the houses, under the beds.

Trees in North Carolina were stable. What could I hold onto in the West? No moss softened the bark of the yucca trees. No lichen inched its way over roots that jutted up from under the earth. No leaves fell in piles as tall as me to cushion a fall, or a jump, or to dissolve into the damp earth as winter approached, coating the ground with slippery softness. I could only cling to the dry desert dust, which slipped through my fingers like breath.

The desert is merciless. It bleaches me, turns my flesh into carrion for the coyote or the turkey vulture. Its sun penetrates everything, leaving no shadow, no shade, no safety. I don't decay here; I fossilize, baked into suspended animation like a tarantula under glass.

At twelve years old, I would have turned back when I saw the bleakness of Texas. I would have gassed up, turned a sharp corner, and returned to the place I knew. We pushed through the wall of sunlight into Arizona and stayed. We kept going west even though no one knew what it was going to be like, if it was going to be a mistake, if we would eventually need to retrace our tracks and go home.

I would have turned back.

When I wrote my first, quite awful, novel, I did turn back. I hit the barren place, the place that offered no light, no hope for what could be in the next chapter, so I decided the book was dead and I abandoned it, a rusted car, along the edge of the interstate. Hope seduced again, and I started a second, also quite awful, novel. I heard the voice of a spider in a prison cell in Salem, Massachusetts, during the seventeenth century. I heard the voice of a woman who had been accused of witchcraft. I found books on the plants and animals of New England. I read up on the burning times. I fell into feminism. Once again, I hit the barren place and abandoned the book.

I wrote my third novel in graduate school, and I had to finish it or I wouldn't graduate. Again, I hit the barren place. But I had a deadline, a workshop group, a student loan. So

I drove through Texas, more because I had to than because I wanted to. I still would have turned back. But because I didn't, I became a writer. I finished a project. I stayed with it when it didn't have anything to say. I stayed with it when its landscape grew gray and sour. I stayed with it while the siren call of another book began its whistle.

There is always a barren place, a place where you feel you don't have enough supplies, or talent, or hope to cross. This is the intersection where hope becomes faith, and you step forward without knowing where you'll end up, with your gallon of water, bottle of sunscreen, and big floppy hat. You step forward because you are establishing trust with the writing. It's waiting to see if you're just a one-night-stand kind of writer, or if you can make a commitment to the long haul.

Step out onto the freeway with a cardboard sign that says WEST and see who stops to pick you up. Someone will because you're standing there, surrendered to the work, surrendered to what you don't know.

## CHAPTER 39

# Disconnection

I confused things with their names: that is belief.

—Jean-Paul Sartre

t's going to happen. You're going to be going full throttle for a week, or a month, or a year, and then—bam! You'll find yourself wondering what on earth you were thinking. You won't recognize your story. Your characters will stop talking to you. You'll realize you started the whole book in the wrong point of view, or the wrong setting, or with the wrong character. You'll sit in front of your computer where previously you've been in blissful harmony with the work, and you'll do nothing. You'll raise your fingers above the keys, pause dramatically in hopes something brilliant will swoop in underneath your fingertips and start writing again, but nothing will happen. You'll suddenly read the World's Most Brilliant Book Just Like the One You're Writing and go order three gallons of Chunky Monkey ice cream to wash it all away. You'll realize that the vampire stories you've been working on diligently for several years are now passé. You'll look to heaven or hell or anywhere in between to find your missing muse. You'll consult old books that once held pearls of wisdom on the writing process only to find them all stupid and irrelevant. You'll walk into your favorite bookstore where you've always found comfort only to see instead a glut of books that no one is buying.

This phase of disconnection hits every writer. Don't make the mistake of taking this phase as the end. Think about it instead like the teenager phase of your book. Remember how fun your kids were when they were teens? Or, if you're not a parent, remember how fun you were as a teen? Yeah. It's coming back to you now, right? The rolling of the eyes. The slamming of the doors. The cries of *no one understands me*. The inability to talk with your mother or father without fighting or crying. The feeling that no one anywhere in the universe has ever been so alone. So different. So strange. So unable to fit into the world you've landed in (not by your own choice, you might add).

Disconnection from your work is not the same as the limbo phase. Limbo is that time between projects when you're not sure where to go next. Disconnection applies to the current project you're working on. You may feel bored with it. You may find yourself vulnerable to seductions from brighter, shinier projects. In short, you and your work don't know how to talk to each other anymore. Where's the writing counselor?

Your book is just going through some growing pains. Its job is to fight with you. To challenge you. To resist the path you've laid out for it. Its job is to wrestle itself free from you so it can find its own voice. Your job during this time is to keep showing up. Remain present. Don't decide you don't love the work anymore. Don't decide to send it off to boarding school. Don't force it to wear a navy blue uniform or take out its piercings. Don't do what every fiber of your being is telling you to do—hold tighter; don't let it get away! No. Stop yourself. Back away. Keep your door open. Keep food in the refrigerator. Don't cut off the bank accounts. This is a critical time in your relationship with your writing. This is the time many a talented writer collapses under the stress of watching what she has loved rebel. It doesn't have to be this way. Patience. Compassion. Kindness. Space. We are cultivating all these qualities with our breathing, shaking, and writing practice.

Don't throw up your hands and walk away. Your work wants to talk to you; it just doesn't know how yet. It needs to find its own identity and then return to you. If you close the door, it can't come back. Keep showing up. Perhaps focus more time now on journaling or prewriting for a different project, but check in every day on this novel. Check in every day on its well-being. "Are you still there? Are you OK? Do you want to talk? Can I get you anything?" And if the answer is no, or if no answers surface at all, return to your desk and keep working. Here's where your maturity and practice will pay off. You'll be able to remain steady while your work goes through its own temper tantrums and identity crises. Your steadfastness will show your writing that you will be there no matter what it does or doesn't do. No matter how easily the words come, or how hard it is to find them. Your love is nonjudgmental. Your compassion endless.

Now at the risk of sounding too Pollyannaish, let me assure you I identify with the frustration of these troubled-teen times. I tend to want to force my work to do something it is (or I am) not yet ready for. I want to do it all *now*. But I have to wait. Don't force. Be steady. Your book will come back to you if you keep the door open. If you keep learning your craft. If you keep showing up. Your book will take you to the next level. Your only task when you feel this disconnection is to step back, keep working, and release your attachment to an outcome. Release your desire for a particular result or a timeline for a particular result.

You're not going to get very far with your daughter if you keep pushing to know her every secret. If you keep following her around on her first dates. If you keep telling her what college program to major in. You're going to create tension and friction between you and your work. You're the writer. Your job is to hold the space. You remain rooted while your work bounces around for a while. You hold the space. There is freedom there.

Don't let yourself fall victim to judgment. Don't tell yourself this wouldn't happen if you were a real writer. A good writer. Even a modestly good writer. This wouldn't happen if you'd planned better. If you hadn't taken that new job. If you didn't just get married. If you didn't just get divorced. If you'd thought your plot through better. If you hadn't tried to mimic another writer's voice. If you hadn't read so many James Bond books before starting. If you'd gotten an MFA. If you hadn't gotten an MFA.

Stop.

Breathe.

Shake.

Pay attention.

1. It's normal to be at odds with your book.
2. It's normal to not like your book.
3. It's normal to feel distant from your book.
4. It's normal to doubt your own ability.

Try to remember what drew you to the book in the first place. You're starting to see why writing is work. Yes, it's fun. Yes, it's fabulous. Yes, it sucks. Yes, it's hard. It's many many things. Sometimes all at the same time. Writing a novel is not like working on an assembly line. One part plot, two parts driving question, one part characterization, throw in a dash of dialogue. Voilá. Story. Nope. Not like that.

You're in the beginning stage. You're birthing your book. You have to step back and let it evolve. Your job—and your only job when writing a first draft—is to write the next right word. Stay present in the body and belly of your story. Resist the urge to leap into the future of your story, or to hold on to past ideas about your story. One word follows the next. This is not new information. It's not new advice. One word plus one word plus one word eventually yields seventy thousand words.

A first novel is often just a first novel. It teaches you how to write a book-length work. It is not the book that you will get published. It is often not even very good. It is the book that teaches you how to be a Writing Warrior. It is the work that is necessary to get you where you ultimately can go. No work is ever wasted. I have many first novels. They all taught me valuable things. I thought they were all going to be the "one." They were not. But they were my companions. And my teachers.

Your job is only to write the next right word.

## CHAPTER 40

# The Mysteries of Fiction

The pages are still blank, but there is a miraculous feeling of the words being there, written in invisible ink and clamoring to become visible.

—Vladimir Nabokov

San Francisco's ghosts are as vibrant as the rainbow flags that fly from the tops of buildings on Market Street. Its ghosts cling to the basement of the Westin St. Francis during the fire after the 1906 quake. They holed up in the wine cellar with a tiny dog, waiting for the rocking and the burning to be over.

The city absorbs everything and everyone. The ruins of the Central Freeway (US Route 101) that collapsed after the '89 Loma Prieta quake have become a green backdrop for the laundromats and hair salons of the newly gentrified Hayes Valley. The city remembers its opium dens and its slave trade in immigrant labor. The city remembers Mark Twain and has yet to forgive him for his "the coldest winter I ever spent was a summer in San Francisco" comment. The city remembers the Beats. North Beach, which isn't what it was, still holds the sound of the pale, white alcoholics who tried to change the world—or at least their perception of the world.

   I walk through the Tenderloin with my friend Dex and
·my husband, Keith. My current novel's protagonist, Helen,
lives there, and I want to get a visceral feel for the neighborhood. Helen is an alcoholic. Her baby, Ellie, drowned at
her breast in 1969. Her daughter, Claire, has just packed up
and moved to god knows where, she thinks somewhere in
Oregon, and her husband, Frank, hasn't come home from
work yet. He hasn't been late coming home in forty years.
She rarely leaves her apartment, which she and Frank have
lived in since the late '60s. Their marriage has become what
many marriages become, a familiarity to be borne with a
Catholic severity. She didn't know she relied on his presence until he didn't return. This night, tonight, June 19,
she is venturing out of her apartment. Forty years from the
day she and Frank first landed in San Francisco and found
themselves in the Haight at a love-in, waiting for the wailing
of Janis Joplin. She is stepping out, presumably to look for
Frank, but even she knows that's only a story she's feeding
herself. She is stepping out to find her city again, the city
that stole her heart, first in the good way, then in the not-
so-good way. The city that broke her on its jagged sidewalks
and crooked streets. The city that still summons her with the
monotonous voice of a Muni railway announcer, *Approach-
ing, outbound, two cars, J, J, in three minutes.* The city that
tricks her into believing she matters, into believing that she
has somewhere to go and someplace to be, simply because
there are so many options for getting places. Who's to know
that when she gets on a train, she only rides from one end to
the other, gets off, and waits for the train to turn around so
she can reboard. She can ride all day like that in the under-
ground. As long as she doesn't come up the stairs into the
light, she could ride forever. She thinks of a snippet of a song
her father sang to her once, something about someone rid-

ing forever through the streets of Boston, but she can't quite remember all the words. Something about the MTA.

My friend Dex is tall, really tall, which is great when you're walking through the Tenderloin at twilight and you're only five feet two. Dex talks to us about the mayor's policy on homelessness. A motel painted baby blue is blockaded with a black gate. There's a sign for a public hearing; the property is to be changed from a tourist motel to a residence inn. A legless man in a wheelchair across the street from us has the shakes. New banners adorn the streetlights: Welcome to Little Saigon. The banners are professional and pastel and don't portray the street we're walking through. The street we're walking down has an occasional open Vietnamese restaurant, a barricaded halfway house.

"Got a light?" asks the skinny man in front of the building.

"You know I don't smoke," says a fat woman, walking into the building. "I tell you that every night."

I try to look without looking. Across the street is a perilously thin woman, her limbs all angles and tattoos. She's pressed into the shoulder of a Latino man, larger, pierced, and laughing. He pulls her across the street. She's wearing black hose that are ripped from knee to crotch. Her skirt is small enough to be a napkin. They touch, this man and this woman; they touch.

People group in fours and fives, rolling dice, pulling out cigarette after cigarette, puffing a few times, before crushing them out on the sidewalk. Hands slip into pockets and into the hands of men who appear and disappear faster than ghosts. The drugs move around us, a river we can choose to step into or step around. All of us feel the pull of the tide.

Does Helen know how close she is to Union Square? Does she know how close she is to the banking centers of the

West Coast? Does she only see 1967? Only see the Haight as it was with the Diggers and the electric light shows and the lost children looking for themselves in tie-dye and glitter? Has she walked down the Haight since Ellie died?

The breath of the Tenderloin is shallow and staccato. It chokes on its inhale and refuses to release all of its exhale. It's getting darker. Shadows move in the park. Where would Helen go out here? Would she see herself reflected in the face of the homeless man who demanded a dime?

A novel has a four-dimensional world. It is not just outlines and ideas in a color- coded computer file. These outlines and ideas form the skin, perhaps. The outer container. But until the book has its own breath, you have only a corpse. It could be a beautifully preserved corpse, with great sentences and perfect punctuation, but until the book breathes on its own, it's dead.

There's a time to build the house for the breath to live in, and there's a time for the breath to enter. Is this breath inspiration? Yes, and no. It's the moment when the soul enters the book. Sometimes it comes early, sometimes after years of waiting. The soul can't come until its time. Don't quit because the work isn't moving quickly enough for you, or because you believe a novel is just constructing the house, one chapter after the next, like laying bricks. The more space you have in your house, the more easily the breath can enter. If you've cemented all the spaces closed with your ideas and directives, it's going to take a pretty strong spirit to slip inside.

Try going outdoors to listen for your book. Maybe even try the shaking practice outdoors! Brenda Ueland, in her book *If You Want to Write*, wrote at length about the importance of walking and writing. When you move your body, you are creating space. Space in your body creates space in your writing. Space in your writing allows for discovery and surprise.

Fiction is, to me, one of the great mysteries of this life. I don't know why particular characters get under our skins; I only know they do in a triumph of imagination and intellect, a union of body, mind, and spirit. Writers come to classes burning with people's voices in their heads, burning with desires. Your characters are part of you. They have chosen you, or you have chosen them; it doesn't matter which way you view the relationship. They're with you. What are you going to do? What are you not going to do?

Treat your characters with respect. They are not pawns for you. They are not mouthpieces for your agendas. They are fleshy and sticky and complicated. They don't always follow Aristotelian arcs. They will show you the story. They will give you their arc. Follow their breathing, not your own. Empathy carries you here. Empathy opens your body to their experiences. Empathy allows you to love them fiercely, no matter what actions they take in the story, no matter what parts of yourself they reflect. Your work will bring you what you need.

"I noticed you don't ever write about your mother," said a questioner from the audience at a recent reading.

That's been true. I have had to keep working through what has been freshest, what has held the most energy. Writing moves energy. Writing makes space.

"My new novel is all about mothers," I say.

And it is, but I don't yet know what form it will take. As writers, it's our job to show up. It's our job to follow a story down false starts and into the streets of the Tenderloin. It's our job to notice when we put our agenda into it, and pull that part out like a bad tooth. It's our job to move into the characters' bodies, minds, and beliefs. Without judgment. Laying down no conditions. Just being ready with a blank page and an empty body.

Just providing space.

## CHAPTER 41

# Tools

The expectations of life depend upon diligence; the mechanic that would perfect his work must first sharpen his tools.

—Confucius

I n the late 1990s, I became obsessed with Frida Kahlo. A few of her paintings came to the Phoenix Art Museum. My best friend and I stood in front of her paintings, almost afraid to speak as we noted the crimson colors, the desperation in the self-portraits, and the dance between love and pain. I watched the 2002 movie *Frida* and decided I wanted to paint my house in the colors of Frida's villa.

My greatest gifts in this life do not revolve around the domestic realm. Cooking, cleaning, gardening—these noble arts don't work well in my world. But what *has* always worked well for me is my intense desire and drive to do something. Once I decide to do something, I will not be deterred.

Off I went to Home Depot, visions of turquoise, yellow, and orange walls dancing in my head. How hard can painting a house be? I bought paint that looked like the colors I wanted. I bought brushes that seemed fun and festive. I bought a drop cloth and a tray and headed home thinking

I could paint the entire house in just a few hours. (I know, I know.)

What I don't do is quit, even when all signs point to: you're being an idiot, Laraine. I had bought the wrong paint (who knew there were so many types of paint and that they all did different things?). I had bought the wrong brushes. I hadn't bought enough paint trays. I had forgotten entirely about something to wash the brushes in. I had no rags. Getting the picture? But I painted. I put on a Bessie Smith CD and I painted into the night. I painted my French doors aqua, but since I had the wrong paint, the paint didn't stick to the door, so I deliberately pulled a lot of it off and called it "distressed." I painted doorframes purple (but neglected to realize the importance of masking off the door knobs and hinges, or, heaven forbid, removing the door knobs and hinges). I splattered paint across my table by accident and proceeded to run my fingers through it to create an artistic table à la first grade finger painting. I got paint on my clothes (yes, no smock) and in my hair. But I was going to finish, and when I did, I ended up with an aqua-yellow-purple mess that I decided I was madly in love with because it was eccentric (just like me). I was not, under any circumstances, going to either (a) start again or (b) pay a professional to come do it right. So I lived for the next few years in a rather eclectic space that in truth didn't convey the message of eccentricity. It conveyed the message of sloppiness, inattention to detail, to be blunt, a half-assed effort.

It was arrogance that took me to Home Depot armed with nothing more than a few childhood paint-by-number horse kits under my belt. It was arrogance that told me that painting was easy, requiring no skill, no craft, no technique. It was arrogance that pushed me through the painting process long after I knew I was in over my head and had no idea what I was doing. And it was arrogance wrapped in denial that allowed me to live in that space so long. When I decided to move, I had to sell the house "as is" because of the disastrous paint job inside. I was unwilling to pay to fix it, even then.

Don't make this mistake with your writing project. Heed the words of choreographer and dancer Twyla Tharp: "Without passion, all the skill in the world won't lift you above craft. Without skill, all the passion in the world will leave you eager but floundering." Respect that your work is a craft. Understand that a hammer is not the only tool in the world, nor is it the tool that will do everything you need. Fiction, poetry, and memoir contain many elements. Your responsibility as a writer is to understand all those elements. What do they do? What can they do for your work? What elements are you strongest with? Weakest with? What do you rely on too heavily? Plotting? Dialogue? Characterization? Language and word choices? Where do you fall short? (Remember, look with soft eyes; be nonjudgmental.) Do an inventory of what you don't know (and this, dear ones, can usually best be done by trying and failing, trying and failing, trying and failing). It's darn difficult to know what you don't know, now isn't it? With each story or poem you write, pay attention to what you thought you wanted to do with it, but found you couldn't. Why couldn't you? Pay attention to where you struggled with the craft. Pay attention to where you struggled with content. Ask questions. Read other poems and stories and ask, How did the author do that? What in that novel filled you with tension? How did the beats work in the dialogue in that short story?

Don't be ashamed of what you don't know. Writing is part intuition, part sound, part instinct. But it is also craft. A committed writer learns all the tools of the craft and knows how and when to use them. She does this by every once in a while painting her house with oil-based paint and watching it peel up at the edges. She does this by more than every once in a while writing a piece that just doesn't work. She does this over and over and over again, until she recognizes what fits and what doesn't. Until her voice emerges strong beneath the craft. Until her craft and all the tools she used to build her work disappear and it looks like she just sat down, picked up a pencil, and wrote. Until it looked like anyone could do it.

## CHAPTER 42

# Rhythm

Everything has rhythm. Everything dances.

—Maya Angelou

A normal human heart's rhythm crescendos and decrescendos in hills and valleys. A normal human heartbeat has peaks of power; it has places to pause; it holds the stillness before the crescendo begins again, and then it holds the thunder-cracking climax at the apex of the hill of electricity. A dead person's rhythm is gone; the line is flat, the energy dispersed. It doesn't matter whether the person died at the peak of power or in the pause; the flat line remains flat. Imagine playing a drum without leaving the space when you lift your hand above its surface. How would you distinguish sound? How would you know how to move your body to the rhythm? How would you distinguish rhythm from noise?

Although there is no single rhythm for a story, all stories have a rhythm. You may think it's exciting to have one car chase scene after another, followed by a murder and a rocket blast-off, but these events, when placed one after the other, form a flat line because they are all peak moments. Tension, that lifeblood of literature, is gone from the work. The extraordinary has become ordinary, and the reader adjusts to chaos as normal. How does one measure the depth of sadness if the entire manuscript has been sad? How does one measure the release of joy if the book has been one long skip through happyland?

Sometimes in yoga class, we'll do an exercise called Laughing Monkey. We lie on our backs with our arms pointed upward and our legs pointed upward. We begin bicycling our legs while using our arms to pull imaginary grapes down from the vines dangling in front of us. Then we're instructed to laugh. First, we have to fake laugh. Then, the instructor will say something like, "Laugh like a witch!" which will result in goofy laughter that may actually result in real laughter. "Laugh like an old man!" "Laugh like a baby!" "Laugh like your mother!" "Laugh like a duck!" "Those of you too serious to laugh, laugh like a banshee!" And so on, all while pumping our arms and legs. The laughter forces oxygen deep into our bellies. The movement creates heat. The churning in our abdomens breaks up stagnation. And laughing of course feels good. It provides a break for people who were trying too hard to form the perfect warrior pose, or for people who were trying too hard to be a bit more flexible today than yesterday. Laughter grounds us. It makes our bodies shake. If you're shaking and writing, your words will form natural slopes and slides, natural peaks and pauses, and the vibrations will tumble them down to the ground.

Remember, you are asking the reader to take a trip with you. Make sure there's time to rest, explore a little, and take an unexpected detour, before resuming the journey. The pointed edge of laughter will make the slice of sorrow that much deeper. Together, there is balance.

CHAPTER 43

# Papa Don't Preach

Arrogance diminishes wisdom.

—Arabian proverb

I n 1986, I drove a two-hundred-dollar 1972 rusted green Buick Century. I had dotted the bumper with feminist bumper stickers until Dad told me to take them off.

"You never know who you might need help from one day," he said. "No reason to make someone angry who could change a tire for you."

I was furious then, scrubbing the bright purple NOW stickers off with a razor blade in the relentless Arizona sun. I had every right to express myself. This was a free country. Billy Joel's "Uptown Girl" blared from the cassette recorder in the driveway. I was in love with Billy Joel. One day he and I would meet and he'd dump Christie Brinkley on the spot. I was as sure of it as I was sure I should use my car as a billboard.

When I first began writing seriously and having my work produced and published, I thought I should (indeed, thought I had an obligation to) use my writing as a bully pulpit. What I discovered pretty quickly was that I wasn't changing anyone's mind about anything. I wasn't opening up the world to a new way of thinking. I was preaching to the choir. Think about it; most people don't go to hear speakers whose views they don't already agree with. So all the shouting, weeping, and gnashing of teeth I thought I was doing for the betterment of mankind fell on the same ears over and over again. I won't deny it felt good to my newly awakened writer's ego to be praised for my "brilliance," but some wiser, far quieter part of me knew I was only shouting, not examining anything deeply or critically. Applause is sweet and seductive, and it's easy to get it when you tell people what they want to hear. But the sweetness dissolves quickly, and you'll find that not only have you become a preacher, but a writer who has been pigeonholed. What if the day arrives in your life (a day you cannot imagine at twenty-two, but I promise will likely come) when you have a change of heart about something you once felt passionately about? Then what? Then your audience no longer receives from you what it expects and turns on you.

I'm not suggesting you avoid exploring issues that are near and dear to you. Indeed, you can't help but do that. I'm not suggesting you ignore controversial issues or avoid making a concrete statement about anything. I am suggesting that when your characters are merely mouthpieces for your viewpoint, readers will spot it right away. Then, if they agree with you, they might carry on reading. If they disagree with you, they'll close the book. Unless you're writing propaganda pieces or actual sermons, leave the moralizing and politicizing to other venues. When readers feel they're getting a message shoved down their throats, they will generally respond by closing off their hearts. Place your characters in situations that are challenging, believable, and full of possibility with no clear right and wrong answers. Then let your characters and the situation duke it out and see how everything changes. Allow readers the space to form their own conclusions about your story's outcome. Your job is to tell the story. Your job is not to implant a particular moral or political agenda.

Leave that to the bumper stickers.

## CHAPTER 44

# Who Hears You First?

Substitute "damn" every time you're inclined to write "very"; your editor will delete it and the writing will be just as it should be.

—Mark Twain

A title is a seduction," said Dad. We were still in Charlotte. I was in the seventh grade, working on my story for the school's short story competition. "A title should have layers of meaning."

I sat on the beige and black tile floor next to his La-Z-Boy chair. He had my typed pages in his hand. I had written about a black cat whose family had moved away and left him. He walked all the way across the country and found them, only to die in the driveway before the family knew he was there.

I wanted to win the competition. This was my first contest, and I'd be the youngest entrant in the field of seventh through ninth graders. Dad had always read my stories first.

"What do you think the story is saying?" he asked.

"That you can't always get what you want."

"What else? What did the cat want?"

"His family."

"And what happened to the cat?"

"He died before he got it."

Dad wrote something on the cover page. "What do you think of this?"

*A Heartbeat from Happiness.*

"They sometimes call the vice president a heartbeat from the presidency," he said. "He's close, but not close enough for it to count. Or you could look at it like there's something as fragile as a heartbeat that could change the course of events. And it has two *h*s in it so it sounds good."

We laughed. I used the title and I won first place in the competition, a construction paper blue ribbon fastened to the front of my orange binder.

My first workshop leader in graduate school told me to stop writing. He told me I had no idea what I was doing. I was in a group with all men, and I had turned in a scene from my novel in which one of the protagonists was raped by her husband. "Men don't do that," he said.

If this man had been the first one to read my work, he might well have been the last. However, I knew he was wrong. I didn't think I had perfected the craft or structure—I knew I still had more to learn—but I also knew he was wrong about my writing. I knew because my first reader had been my dad, and I knew because I had been writing as long as I could hold a pencil and that I loved writing more fiercely than anything. One teacher's opinion could not alter that love. This was an extremely valuable experience for me, though. I learned to trust myself first—not blindly in the "everything I write is brilliant" way, but in the solid, rooted "I am a writer" way. I hadn't defended that person in me before, and it was important for my career that I do so.

I am always the first reader of my work. The reading must be done with unconditional love. Not blind love, not obsessive love, not jealous, angry love. Detached love. With an eye that sees beauty even under a deformity. An eye that loves enough to prune what is choking the vine and to water what is dying. When I have shaped a work to the best of my ability, given my own blinders, I let it go to others who see with fierce and brilliant love the heartbeat of the work.

Choose your early readers carefully. They must respect the craft. They must respect the story, and they must respect you. If they love you from a place of ego, it will not work. If they are envious of you, it will not work. If they want to be you, it will not work. If they are frustrated writers, it will not work. An early reader must step aside and step into the work in front of them. An early reader must hold your work like a newborn kitten, amazed at both the delicate nature of its precious young life and at the awesome potential of the full-grown work. An early reader must see both. When you find yours, you will have found the greatest treasure in your writing life.

## CHAPTER 45

# Loneliness

I live with the people I create, and it has always
made my essential loneliness less keen.

—Carson McCullers

T here's no way around the fact that writing is a solitary
activity. Yes, you can go to classes. You can join critique groups. You can lurk in writing forums online
and read writing blogs. You can hang out in bookstores and
cool coffee shops and libraries. But you will realize at some
point in your career that peace with being alone is key to
your ability to write well and consistently.

I wish I could be pithy and cute here, but I can't be.
There's you and your work, and whether you dress it up and
take it out to Starbucks or Martha's Vineyard or a Super 8
Motel in a tiny town in Kansas, there's only you and your
work. Your critique group mates can only take you so far.
Your teacher can only go with you so far. You'll never know
what you're made of until you sit long enough with the writing to move through the pulls for companionship (whether
virtual or "real"). How long can you sit still before you check
your e-mail? Your cell phone? A website? These are ways of

reaching out to the world (and that's an important thing), but they are also ways of distracting you from your work.

I don't feel lonely when I'm working. I feel the loneliness when I am avoiding working, when I'm distracting myself from the story or essay. When I am distracted, I've let my mind move in and take over. When I'm in the flow of the story, there's no room for distraction. My characters feed me like friends, and they demand my time like relationships.

The writer's loneliness is strongest when we feel we're most separated from our work. Remember that you created that separation. You can tear it down. Use your tools—your breathing, shaking, and writing practices. These tools help prevent the wall between you and your work from going up in the first place. These tools help maintain your balance, your open energy channels—in short, your flow. When you're in flow, you realize there's no separation in the universe. When you forget you're in flow, you suffer with ideas of loneliness, fear, and tension. It really is the writing practice that keeps you in motion. The consistency of showing up for your work that eases the suffering of loneliness.

Yes, you may be alone in your room writing. But you are connected to everything, every writer who is currently writing or who has written in the past. Every ancestor in your lineage. The animals and plants that have nurtured you. You are part of the continuum, not an isolated part watching on the riverbank. You contain everything within you that you will ever need.

Just sit still long enough to uncover it.

## CHAPTER 46

# Betrayals

It's always our touches of vanity
That manage to betray us.

—Christopher Fry

So here's the good news. You can't betray what you don't care about. Here's the not-so-good news. You only betray the ones you love. This betrayal is going to happen in your relationship with your writing. At least once. Probably more than once because the first few times you're not going to realize what it is. You're going to call it something else, like writer's block, or busy-ness, or family obligations. You might call it laziness, or falling in love, or a change in priorities. But what's happened is that you've betrayed your writing in some way.

Here's more good news. Writing is very forgiving when you step up to the plate and make amends. However, writing is very vengeful when you don't acknowledge what has happened.

Don't stop reading now. I know this may sound a touch more punitive than you would like. Hang with me for a story.

I worked for a time at a local black box theatre in Phoenix called Planet Earth Multicultural Theatre. It was a warehouse theatre in the part of town no woman went without her mace. I spent most evenings there, after working my nine-to-five job in a different part of town. I would pack a peanut butter and jelly sandwich and a slew of Diet Cokes and settle in to the theatre/gallery space where I first heard my work performed. I was a playwright-in-residence there for a few years, and I taught some classes in playwriting and fiction writing. I was learning the craft of writing. I was learning how to be a teacher. I was learning just exactly how badly I wanted to write.

Many opportunities presented themselves to quit, not the least of which was the nineteen- and twenty-hour days I was putting in between the theatre and my "real" job. I loved sitting in the Goodwill-find chairs, watching the actors and director rehearse my plays. I loved rewriting on the spot when I heard the lines fumble in the actors' mouths. I loved the actors' input into the characters' development, but I'll be honest, I really loved it when audiences would come and want to talk to the playwright. *Yes, yes, it was me. Yes, I am young. Oh, twenty-four. Oh, thank you! I'm so glad you enjoyed it.* My ego loved it. Loved it, loved it, loved it, and true to an ego's job, it wanted more. When the opportunity arrived to sell a script to a director I respected, I jumped at the chance. It was a small sum, just one hundred dollars and a 15 percent share of the door, but it was the most money I'd ever earned off my writing, and I was sure I was well on my way to the career I'd always known was coming.

At first, everything was fine. I had input in casting and was happy. Before long though, I watched my script turn into something I didn't recognize. The director (as directors do) had his own opinion about the play's direction. He had his own vision of the arc he wanted to see and the themes he wanted to emphasize. Today, I look back and I have no idea why I thought someone would reproduce my play verbatim.

It just doesn't happen that way for anyone. I watched the way the director was cutting the play. The way he was rewriting. The way he was taking what seemed like only the names of my characters and turning them into something unrecognizable. For a hundred dollars.

Selling your work is selling your work, whether you get one hundred dollars or one hundred million dollars. Maybe it goes down a little better for a hundred million dollars. I don't know. The play went on. People came. And as I stood in the lobby, people who had come to see my other shows came up to me. I could tell they weren't quite sure what to say. Finally, "It just didn't sound like you," they'd say. Or, "It wasn't quite what I was expecting." Yeah. I knew it as it was happening. The play was no longer mine, and I didn't fight for it because I had my hundred dollars in hand. The work was no longer mine. I was new to this game. I was trying to be professional. I also, back to the ruthless honesty part of this deal, wanted to avoid confrontation more than I wanted to defend my writing. This was the betrayal. Not the selling of it, but the lack of defending it. This was where I turned my back on my work, and this is when the rift between us began.

Sold work gets reworked all the time. Novels are adapted to films, and the novelist hangs her head. She can't recognize her story, but she sold her book. It's what we do. If you want to retain all your rights to your work, don't publish it in any traditional way. But if you do sell your work, then other people will be involved. That's the way it goes. It'll be a director or an editor. It'll be an actor or a producer. It'll be someone, and they have a right to get involved because you agreed to the process. So you have to learn what battles to fight and what battles to let go. You have to learn when it's an ego response (sounds like: *No! All my words are perfect and brilliant and untouchable. You, mere mortal, can never expect to understand what I was trying to do. Perhaps you should go back*

to being a dishwasher in lower Manhattan. *Out of my sight!*).
And you have to learn when the response comes from resistance and laziness (sounds like: *Oh wow. Yeah. I knew that
part wasn't really working. But do you know how much work
it's going to take to fix it? That's going to require rewriting the
entire first act and, honestly, I don't care so much anymore.*). And
you have to learn when the response is working *in service to*
the greater good of the work. This happens when the ego
steps out of the way. It happens when you are able to get out
of your own way and recognize that the input of others can
make your work better than it could be on its own. It happens when you can hear what's being said, can recognize
what's of value in what's being said, and are prepared to take
the necessary action to integrate the suggestions.

This doesn't mean you're a doormat, taking every single
piece of feedback and slapping it all together in a smorgas-
bord of ideas and directions. It's your work, no matter what
you were paid for it. But there are compromises every writer
must make, and those compromises are generally for the
greater good of the work. I field a lot of questions from students about editors. They tend to think one of two things:
the editor will completely rewrite the work and fix everything
the writer was too lazy to fix (grammar and spelling!), or the
editor is some kind of power freak who wants to take the
writer's talent and spin it in some horrific way. Neither of
these fall anywhere close to my experience.

Students often don't want to submit their work for publication because they're afraid they will lose their voice if
someone else gets hold of it. A good editor helps you make
your own voice better. The editor doesn't take away your
voice and turn it into someone else's or her own. For this
relationship to work, however, you have to be open to hearing someone make comments about your work. You have to
be open to changing the way you initially approached some-

thing. (Sometimes their ideas are better, sometimes not, but the way you choose to respond to these suggestions will speak volumes about you as a writer.) Respond with courtesy. Digest the comments. Ask yourself: Will this make my work better? Is this something I never considered? Why is this comment coming up now? What did I forget to say? Where was I unclear? Editors want to help you and help your work. Let them.

Accepting feedback is not a betrayal of your work. Sometimes, though, your work does become discombobulated and you find you no longer recognize it. There may be nothing you can do about it, depending on the kind of contract you've entered into. You may have to follow this to the end, watching your vision crumble. But you may have options, such as paying back your advance and pulling the work (this may have longer term consequences for your career than you realize at this point, so think long and hard first). You may be able to renegotiate the deadlines so that you can rewrite with a different focus. Every choice you make will have consequences; sometimes it's right to walk away and cut your losses, and sometimes it's right to stay and fight. Practice self-observation without judgment. Be ruthlessly honest with yourself. There are no absolute answers here.

In my situation with the play, I could have fought more for my work. I could have argued with the director. I never presented my concerns to him. I was too wrapped up in who this director was (I thought he was untouchable in the local community). I was afraid that if I challenged him he would never produce my work again. I was also afraid that maybe he was right and I had made some serious miscalculations about what the work was supposed to be. I was too inexperienced to know the difference between my intuition and my ego response. It takes time to learn the difference, and I'll bet there will always be a bit of confusion. Ego tends to be louder than intuition.

Ego tends to respond with contraction and reaction. Intuition feels softer, more spacious. *Wait; wait. That's not quite right.* That's a different response from: *He's destroying my genius!* As you get more practice watching your behavior in situations, you'll become more skilled at determining who inside of you is speaking.

I didn't stand up for my work. I could have and I should have. It wasn't like I'd sold a screenplay and Johnny Depp had signed. This was a low stakes theatre. A low stakes production. But I remained silent. That was the betrayal. The betrayal wasn't whether or not I stood up for it or didn't. The betrayal wasn't in the outcome. The betrayal was that I knew what the right thing to do was, yet did nothing.

That was the last play I produced at that theatre. Not because I had burned bridges, but because I couldn't write. I couldn't find a way back to plays, a way back to drama and the stage. I had betrayed my writing, and my muse turned her back on me. I didn't know that was what was happening. I didn't understand the sacred relationship between a writer and the writing. I was still exclusively an ego-based writer. I still thought I was in charge of the whole thing. I thought I could turn it on and off like a light switch. I thought I dictated the terms and conditions of its arrival.

In negotiations with your work, fight the fights that matter. Maintain a consistent relationship with your writing so it doesn't think you've turned away. Remember that you are in a partnership, not in a mistress/servant relationship. What would you do in the same situation if your writing were a person? Or if your writing was yourself, because ultimately, of course, what you do or do not do to and for your writing, you do to and for yourself.

How do you want to be treated? How do you want to be remembered? How do you want to love?

## CHAPTER 47

# Natural Talent

Use what talents you possess; the woods would be
very silent if no birds sang there except those that
sang best.

—Henry van Dyke

I t happens every semester. The student creeps up to you
in the very last breath of your office hour. Or she waits
until the rest of the class has gathered up their backpacks
and water bottles. Sometimes he's shy. Sometimes she's bold.
Sometimes he poses it as a challenge. Sometimes more of a
prayer.

"Do I have any talent?"

For a writing teacher, this question is the equivalent of
being asked to reveal state secrets to the Taliban. And, fortunately, I've honed my Special Forces resistance skills over
the years to where I can keep a poker face and provide the
only answer that is ethical: "I can't answer that."

The reason the poker face is needed is because I'm still a
human being. The students I work with present a wide range
of abilities. I have personal tastes that I try to keep out of the
classroom, but they are still part of how I see literature.

I'm convinced that people ask the question because they want to be validated. My job is not to validate. My job is to help my students grow as writers. Think about it. The last time you asked someone if your butt looked fat in those jeans, did you really want them to say, "Actually, yes it does"? Likely not.

I am not the Talent Police, nor am I the Talent Judge. But talent isn't all that matters. Perseverance, a commitment to learning the craft, writing writing writing writing writing, studying grammar, reading reading reading reading reading—these things can make a writer successful. I can't even tell you with certainty whether or not a piece can be published. So much of publishing is changing and out of our control that we can't possibly say with definitive authority, No, it'll never make it, or, Yes! It's a best seller. No one knows these things. Please don't ask us. Ask questions such as, "Who can I read more of to learn more about plot?" or "What are some of the different ways I could have approached that character conflict?" or "Where do you think the work fell into cliché?" Ask concrete developmental questions about your work. We can answer those. The work will improve. And the rest will go where it will go.

I think of talent as a magic bean. All of us received a handful of magic beans, but none of us got the same assortment of magic beans. All of these magic beans were not programmed to sprout at the same time. Sometimes they lie dormant until the circumstances arise for them to bloom. Sometimes they are nurtured from early childhood. Some people publish a book in their early twenties. Others not until their eighties. Everyone didn't get the same set of circumstances, so talent cannot be measured in an Excel spreadsheet. Talent can't be ranked, quantified, or implanted.

I also know that since all people are not given equal gifts, all people cannot accomplish the exact same things. No matter how much I want to be a blues singer, it just ain't happening in this life. That doesn't mean I can't enjoy music and singing, but it means the open mic or karaoke night is as far as I'm going to get with my musical ability.

If you're in my class, I'll never tell you whether I think you're talented enough because I can't know. I will tell you if individual sentences, or stories, or poems sing. I will tell you how to make a piece stronger.

Do your own writing. Study. Read. Read. Read. Write. Read. Push yourself. Don't get complacent (oh, I already know how to write dialogue). I'll bet there's something new you could learn. Be a constant student whether you're in class or not. Be in service to your art. Listen to it. Walk with it. That's the relationship that will get you wherever you and your writing are supposed to end up in this crazy world.

But talent? Don't worry about it. Your job is to use the magic beans you've been given to the best of your ability. Don't waste them comparing your beans to everyone else's beans. Your commitment is to your growth with your art. Nothing more and nothing less is required of you.

You may never be able to string together clauses like Faulkner, but that's OK. We've had one Faulkner. What is it that you can do?

CHAPTER 48

# Spiral Dance

And those who were seen dancing were thought
insane by those who could not hear the music.

—Friedrich Nietzsche

N ovelist Ursula K. Le Guin decries the linear perspective that dominates modern storytelling. She
says it's "like an arrow, starting here and going
straight there and THOK! hitting its mark." Furthermore,
she complains, modern plots are usually advanced through
conflict, as if interesting action can't possibly arise from any
other catalyst.

This week, in an introductory creative writing class, we
began in-class writing at last, and I started the inevitable and
constant work of helping students look inward with ruthless
scrutiny and ruthless compassion. Much of what I teach is
not about writing in a linear way. Most of what I do is guide
students into their lifetime journey of self-exploration. Until
they look inside themselves and find themselves shocked
and awed, in despair and in love with what they see, they will
not be able to create believable worlds on the page.

I walk around the classroom and listen to their disclaim-
ers of their work. Before they'll share what they wrote, they

tear it down. New work is as fragile as an antique teacup. New work must be allowed to breathe and speak before the craftsperson shapes it. One student mentioned that she wanted to develop a more sacred relationship with her writing. I rarely hear that during the first few weeks, but by the end of a semester with me, few people believe writing is anything but a sacred relationship.

Le Guin's statement hits at the heart of my philosophy on writing. Yes, plot is a causal relationship, but the structure of a story or a book can be anything but linear and expected. This event may follow that event in your "real life," but in narrative you have the luxury of manipulating time and space. Pearl S. Buck says, "One faces the future with one's past." We look ahead to what we can be and do based on where we have been and what we have done. So even "real life" is not as directly causal as it appears on the surface. This follows that because of that and that and that, or because that and that and that did *not* occur, this did. It's not a line. Remove a section within a line and you've still got a line. Remove a piece of a spiral and the whole pattern changes.

Whether my students publish or not, writing a novel or a story and following it through revisions, critique sessions, self-doubts, false praise, and finally that cutting, compassionate eye from within will change them forever. The world is a better place with each story written. Every time you take a risk with your work, you give yourself the ability to take more risks in your "regular" life. The way you approach your writing is the way you will approach your life. Discipline and compassion cannot be turned on and off.

When I look back on my life, I do not see it as a journey from point A to point B. I see it in defining moments. I see it in overlapping memories and overlapping relationships. I see it in a merging between what happened and what I wanted to have happened and what I have subsequently told myself happened. And I hope, when I am reflecting on my life for the final time, I will see the pattern I have written.

My pattern will not be a line that stretches from birth to death. My pattern will be a series of spirals, of turning in and back and around and forward. My pattern will dance, even as I spin away.

This is my sincerest wish for my students and for you. When you look back on your lives, may your patterns spin and twist and meander. May the ending be the only possible conclusion to the work you've done. May you close your eyes and whisper, "It is perfect," and spin away.

# THE WRITING WARRIOR PRACTICE

An ounce of practice is worth more than tons of preaching.

—Mahatma Gandhi

Part 5, Deepening Your Writer's Roots, gave you some insights into the mysterious side of the writing process. This mystery is awe-inspiring and often frustrating. The more you understand the ways writing can manifest in your life, the less likely you'll be to throw up your hands and walk away. Every writer walks his or her own path. Understanding some of the common pitfalls along the path will help you avoid succumbing to them.

Writing goes through phases. Sometimes we're intimate with it. Sometimes we're detached from it. Sometimes we can't figure it out at all. Remember the concept of impermanence. The next time you sit down to write will be different from this time. Trust that nothing will be the same from day to day. Rather than be unsettled by that, let it be grounding. You'll be lonely sometimes. You'll doubt yourself and your work. You'll wonder if you have enough talent or discipline or passion. Keep showing up. Each word follows the word before it, just like each breath follows the previous one. You don't have to know where you're going to end up somewhere wonderful.

When the mystery becomes uncomfortable or unfamiliar, return to the familiarity and stability of the Writing Warrior practice. Anchor yourself with your breath and your pen. Move through your discomfort with shaking. Tomorrow will be different from today. Approach each writing session with emptiness and acceptance for what arises. Your relationship with writing is not static; it is constantly evolving with each stroke of your pen. Let it grow as you do, ever more free, light, and awake.

## INTERNAL CONVERSATIONS

*You can use these internal conversation exercises for personal work. The deeper your relationship with yourself, the deeper your writing becomes. Feel free to use poetry or prose to respond.*

Create a chronology of your relationship with writing. Do you remember when you first met? How would you describe that relationship over time?

What/who has haunted you? What are your obsessions? How have they manifested in your writing?

Examine your writing process. What gifts has writing given you? When/how have you been surprised by what writing has to offer? When/how have you been frightened by it? Enthralled with it?

When/how have you experienced "limbo" in your writing? What does that in-between place feel like? Be specific. Find an image to represent limbo for you.

What projects have you started and been unable to finish? Are any of them worth revisiting with fresh eyes?

What ghosts or representations of yourself could you pick up alongside the road? What might they whisper to you if they could?

How does the Texas phase manifest for you? Can you come up with another metaphor that's more accurate for your experience? How many times have you turned back from or stopped writing a project? Observe without judgment. Do any of those projects still have energy for you?

What have you learned about yourself from each of your projects or characters? Take time for gratitude.

Have you ever betrayed your writing? Take time now to acknowledge and write about that experience. What did you lose? What did you gain? What did you learn?

How would you describe your relationship to solitude? You might like to think of solitude as a companion rather than an adversary. What can it teach you? What can it show you about yourself? What do you fear or avoid about it? What do you welcome about it?

---

WRITE NOW

*The following exercises can be applied to works in progress or used as prewriting. Feel free to use poetry or prose to respond.*

Keep a journal just for characters, voices, and snippets. It is very easy for these brief, critical bits of the writing process to get lost if they're randomly written down on sticky notes or napkins. You might call this journal "The Gathering Place."

Take a scene or chapter from a work in progress and examine its rhythm. Start with the big picture things. Pay attention to each scene's pacing. How much action is there?

How much lingering? Are the right things moving quickly? Are you devoting enough time to key moments of change? How is the rhythm overall? Is there room for the reader to breathe, or is everything at a manic pace? Next, examine each sentence's rhythm. This is best done by reading them aloud. Is everything staccato? Too long? Notice any repetitions with vowel sounds or consonants? If so, do you like the way that sounds or can you change it? Listen for the music not just of the entire book, but also of each sentence.

Comb through your work for any signs of preaching. When you come across a character or scene with an agenda in it that *does not serve the story* (the key is the story, not your own personal morals or beliefs), cut it. If you simply can't cut it, then explore your characters more fully to find a way to incorporate the scene without having your agenda in it. Generally, a deeper exploration of a character will reveal the humanity in all of your characters. Once the human connection is established, it's harder to be judgmental in your work. It's harder to label something good or evil once we understand the motivations behind who is doing the actions.

Do you have a writing group or partner? If not, how can you find one in your community? The community college or local bookstore is a great place to start. There are also lots of online writing communities. Be as willing to provide honest, compassionate feedback as you are eager to receive it. It will likely take a while to find a group or a person you truly connect with, but it is worth the search.

Where can you deepen your understanding of your craft? Do you struggle with plot? Dialogue? Creating tension? Pacing? Seek out not just books on writing, but works of fiction, poetry, and creative nonfiction to study from the perspective of a writer, not a reader. Be careful of feeling like you've "arrived." There is always something more to learn, to read, and to try. Don't solidify in a sense of achievement. Be willing to start something brand new.

Make a list of twelve books you've always wanted to read. Read one book per month from the eye of a writer, not a reader. Don't give up on the book midway through. Stick with it until the end. Remember: you do not have to like a book to learn from it. Find something amazing about the craft choices in each book. Find something connected to writing that you could learn more about and incorporate into your own work. Continually ask *how* did the author achieve that? *Why* did the author choose that method? *What* did the author gain by those choices? *What* did the author lose?

Create a commitment plan between you and your writing. Only you can make yourself write. Not me. Not a class. Not a book. Only you. What vows can you write to each other to ensure a lifelong Writing Warrior relationship?

# About the Author

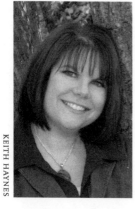

KEITH HAYNES

LARAINE HERRING holds an MFA in creative writing and an MA in counseling psychology. She has developed numerous workshops that use writing as a tool for healing. She is the author of *Writing Begins with the Breath: Embodying Your Authentic Voice; Lost Fathers: How Women Can Heal from Adolescent Father Loss;* the novel *Ghost Swamp Blues;* and the short story collection *Monsoons.* Her short stories, poems, and essays have appeared in national and local publications. Her fiction has won the Barbara Deming Award for Women, and her nonfiction work has been nominated for a Pushcart Prize. She currently teaches creative writing in Prescott, Arizona.

Learn more about Laraine at www.laraineherring.com. Check out videos related to writing and the concepts in this book on her YouTube.com channel.